HOW TO:
UNDERSTAND, CHOOSE CARE FOR, AND MANAGE SCOLIOSIS

The Scoliosis Coach Handbook
Written by: Dr. Andromeda Stevens, D.C.

This book details the author's personal experiences with, and opinions about, scoliosis. The author is not your healthcare provider. The author and publisher are providing this book and its contents on an "as is" basis and make no representations or warranties of any kind concerning this book or its contents. The author and publisher disclaim all such representations and warranties, including for example warranties of merchantability and healthcare for a particular purpose. In addition, the author and publisher do not represent or warrant that the information accessible via this book is accurate, complete, or current. The statements made about products and services have not been evaluated by the U.S. Food and Drug Administration. They are not intended to diagnose, treat, cure, or prevent any condition or disease. Please consult with your physician or healthcare specialist regarding the suggestions and recommendations made in this book. Except as specifically stated in this book, neither the author nor publisher, nor any authors, contributors, or other representatives will be liable for damages arising out of or in connection with the use of this book. This is a comprehensive limitation of liability that applies to all damages of any kind, including (without limitation) compensatory, direct, indirect, or consequential damages; loss of data, income, or profit; loss of or damage to property and claims of third parties. You understand that this book is not intended as a substitute for consultation with a licensed healthcare practitioner, such as your physician. Before you begin any healthcare program or change your lifestyle in any way, you should consult your physician or another licensed healthcare practitioner to ensure that you are in good health and that the examples contained in this book will not harm you. This book provides content related to physical and/or mental health issues. As such, the use of this book implies your acceptance of this disclaimer.

Library of Congress Control Number: 2022917023
ISBN: 979-8-9866508-2-1 Paperback
ISBN: 979–8–9866508-3-8 E-book

U.S. Copyright Office
101 Independence Ave. S.E. Washington, D.C. 20559-6000
1-9190306091

Dr. Andromeda Stevens, DC
16430 Ventura Blvd Suite 108, Encino, CA 91436
@ScoliosisCoach
www.ScoliosisCoach.com
https://linktr.ee/scoliosiscoach
Facebook https://www.facebook.com/ScoliosisCoach
Instagram https://www.instagram.com/scoliosiscoach/
Vimeo https://vimeo.com/scoliosiscoach
YouTube youtube.com/c/ScoliosisCoach
Yelp https://www.yelp.com/biz/andromeda-stevens-dc-schroth-scoliosis-coach-encino

ISBN 979-8-9866508-3-8

90000 >

9 798986 650838

SCOLIOSIS COACH

ISBN 978-0-99-702549-1

90000

9 780997 025491

Bar Code E-book

Bar Code Paperback

SCOLIOSIS COACH HANDBOOK INDEX

ACKNOWLEDGMENTS

I want to personally recognize the people who contributed to this work.

Ray Diaz, of SoCal Scoliosis Care, Phillip P. Ambroset, C.P.O. of OP in Motion, Gez Bowman of LA Brace, and Dr. Fred Edelman, MD.

To Erin O'Bryan for her contribution to the nutrition chapter of this book and Lauren Higginson for her contribution to the psychology and resources chapters.

To Dr. Gazmarian, MD, Dr. Marc Moramarco, DC, and Dr. Hans Weiss, MD, and Nikos Karavidas for their mentorship and camaraderie in the field of scoliosis care.

I would like to thank Cherry Trumbull and Glenn Stevens for their endless support and assistance in the editing of this book.

Finally, I thank my patients, their parents, and their families for the trust they have placed in me, for the opportunity to learn from them, and for the inspiration to write this book.

PROLOGUE/PREFACE

I would like to tell you my scoliosis story. When I was a young girl around 10-12 years old, I had upper back pain which was pretty persistent. Sometimes, the pain was acute. I remember keeping it from my parents and just coping with it. There would be many days that I would wake up in pain and have pain all day at school. It would feel better to lean forward onto my desk and rest or to extend backward over my chair and "crack" my back. I did not know I was making it worse. I will tell you more about that later. One day my mother and I were running around the house playing tag and just generally goofing off. I snuck up quickly behind her and surprised her by tapping her on the back. It startled her so badly, that she whiplashed her neck. She then began regular visits to a chiropractor, Dr. Renee Stampler, D.C., in Beverly Hills, California. My mother would take me with her most of the time. During one visit, Dr. Stampler took a look at me and discovered that I had scoliosis. She began adjusting me and I continued using chiropractic as a way of managing my pain over the years. As I grew older I also started doing lots of massage work for the pain.

Dr. Stampler set a positive example and inspired me to enroll in chiropractic college. Unfortunately, my professors never discussed scoliosis or anything about muscular work. My coursework was purely structural and clinical work. I took a hiatus from chiropractic college to go to massage school to learn more about healing work, muscles, touch and breathing. This was a very interesting break from my college experience. As the years went by, my pain would come and go but much of the time pain would be the very first thing I felt when I woke up and the very last thing I felt before going to sleep. Sometimes it drove me crazy. While I was in my last term of chiropractic college, we all had to work in the clinic and get X-rays to assess each other. My scoliosis was

5

pretty mild and only in the upper part of my back but for whatever reason, it caused me substantial pain. Years later I was running a chiropractic clinic and a Pilates studio in Los Angeles and had a client come to me with a question. She had severe scoliosis at 50+ years of age and was being told it was time to have surgery. She was horrified and asked if there was anything else that I knew of that she could try. I did some research and found a clinic on the outskirts of Los Angeles that did something called the "Schroth Method". I sent her to investigate the technique and she took one of my Pilates instructors along with her for a weekend "boot camp" style of treatment. They came back with a very interesting handbook of exercises, which although it was not customized to the client, aroused my curiosity.

I started investigating Schroth and found a doctor in Massachusetts named Dr. Marc Moramarco, D.C., who was interested in coming to Los Angeles to see some of his patients. We agreed that he would use my office as a meeting place. He saw patients and I watched and followed along. I jumped in as a patient and performed the Schroth exercises for the better part of four hours over a 24 to 48-hour period. I was so sore I was flabbergasted. I was working muscles I had not worked in years, shifting my curve and breathing in areas of my rib cage that were not normally accessed. I continued the exercises and protocols and to my astonishment, my pain dropped down to near zero. I started trying to figure out how I could get certified in this methodology. I was repeatedly rejected by various schools that didn't believe that chiropractors should be practicing the Schroth method! Can you imagine? A practitioner who deals with nothing but spines all day is being told that she has no business using the Schroth method! I was bewildered, frustrated and mad. I persisted and found out that Dr. Moramarco was working with Dr. Hans Rudolph Weiss who is a grandson of the Schroth family and was coming to the United States to present the first program in the U.S.A. I jumped at the opportunity and booked my ticket to Massachusetts. The course was intense and extraordinary.

I started slowly implementing the program with a few clients and learned and practiced and studied and asked lots of questions of my mentors. My practice grew and I rented more space. I then traveled back to Massachusetts for the level II Schroth program. Having been a chiropractor and Pilates instructor by this point for the better part of 23+ years, I saw so many Pilates instructors struggle with clients who had scoliosis and were not seeking treatment anywhere else other than the Pilates studio or had received unhelpful treatment. Instructors would continually ask me what they could be doing to help their clients and I was perplexed at how to assist them in helping others although they were not clinicians. I started to take every Pilates-based scoliosis workshop and read every scoliosis, Pilates, and yoga manual that I could find. I took many in-person and online workshops. They all seemed to contradict my Schroth training in one way or another or were simply inappropriate for a Pilates instructor. It was clear that untold numbers of instructors worldwide were following these protocols and possibly making things worse for their clients.

I set out to create a manual for Pilates teachers that would supply them with enough helpful information about what to do and more importantly, what not to do with a scoliosis client while reaming within the scope of the teacher's practice. This has been an extraordinarily rewarding project. Meanwhile, in my private practice, I was mostly working with individuals who were adults and had been suffering from scoliosis their whole lives without much success treatment-wise. I worked with parents of children who were newly diagnosed, completely overwhelmed and frankly, freaked out. They had so many questions and concerns and sometimes had been given conflicting information. I thought it was time to write down the basics, whether for persons with scoliosis or parents trying to help their child navigate this confusing new landscape.

My sincere hope is that my experience and knowledge will help you with your situation. Please feel free to reach out to me personally to discuss any questions you may have.

ABOUT THE AUTHOR

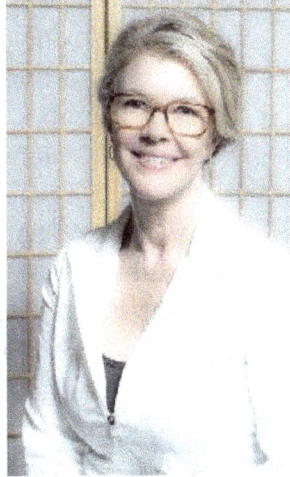

Dr. Andromeda Stevens, D.C. prompted by her scoliosis, became a chiropractor and has been practicing since 1996. Andromeda was introduced to Pilates in the early '90s and was so inspired that she became a Pilates Method Alliance Gold Certified Teacher™ (13657 PMA# OR 10112 NPCT#). The profound results with her patients, as well as the inability to find quality Pilates Instructors for the Studio, led her to co-found Pilates Sports Center in 2000, with Kelli Altounian in Los Angeles. To train instructors in the method, The Pilates Sports Center Pilates Teacher Training Program, the Burn at the Barre Teacher Training Program and the Pilates Master Teacher Program are now taught worldwide with the mission of providing the highest standard of excellence in Pilates education. The practice specializes in treating scoliosis using the Schroth Method. Dr. Stevens is Level II Schroth certified by Dr. Hans R. Weiss, M.D. (the grandson of K. Schroth) and she is one of very few certified in the U.S.A. in the original method.

Credentials:
Graduate – Cleveland Chiropractic College of Los Angeles 1996
Schroth Best Practice® Level I & II Certified by Dr. Hans-Rudolf Weiss, M.D. and Dr. Marc Moramarco, D.C. USA: Schroth Best Practice Academy
Certification Course on BSPTS-Concept by Rigo Basic Level
Course on Scoliosis and Spinal Disorders
PSSE Schroth Certified – Nikos Karavidas

Postgraduate certification: Cox® Technic - Flexion/Distraction Technique for treatment of discs

Cupping Therapy Trained

National Pilates Certification Program (NPCP) "Gold" Certified Teacher™ National Pilates Certification Program

Integrated Flexibility Training – The Sports Club/LA

BalletCore® Certified

Massage Therapist – Touch Therapy Institute

Graduate of Advances in Pilates – Long Beach Dance Conditioning

Co-Founder of Pilates Sports Center International, Inc.

Co-Creator of the PSC Pilates Teacher Training Program

Co-Creator of the PSC International Master Training Program

Co-Creator of Pilates Sports Centers Burn at the Barre™ Teacher Training Programs (Level I & II)

Co-Produced and Created over 14 digital titles

Co-Wrote or Co-created over 19 workshops

Co-Creator and Presenter: Pilates Expo Los Angeles

Presenter: Mad Dogg WSSC / MindBody Fit-Pro Conference / Balanced Body Pilates On Tour / Inner Idea Conference / Body Mind Spirit Expo / Human Movement Conference / Pilates On Tour / PMA Conferences / Higgy Bears Higgy Con

Master Teacher Trainer for Reebok Sports Club NY 2007

Pilates Method Alliance Registry of Teachers

Participant: PMA Fostering Future Professionals Program

PMA Approved Schools List

CEC Provider NCPT

Board of Directors – The Pilates Initiative

Multiple Workshops were completed with Jay Grimes, Kathy Corey, Rael Isacowitz, Mary Bowen, Lolita San Miguel, Ron Fletcher, Cara Reeser, Alan Herdman, Mari Winsor and many more.

Author of Scoliosis Coach Handbook

www.ScoliosisCoach.com

1. WHAT IS SCOLIOSIS?

Scoliosis is a side (lateral) curvature and twisting of the spine. The spine may curve from side to side, forming an "S" or a "C" shape, rather than a straight line. The term Scoliosis comes from the Greek: skoliōsis meaning "crooked" or twists and turns.

As the spine curves sideways, the individual bones (vertebrae) also twist, like the steps of a spiral staircase, around the vertical axis of the spinal column. As these bones twist, the ribs that are attached to them also rotate and may create a "bump" or prominence on the back. This is usually the first "telltale sign" of scoliosis noticed by a parent or a physician. This rib prominence is usually what cosmetically bothers a person the most.

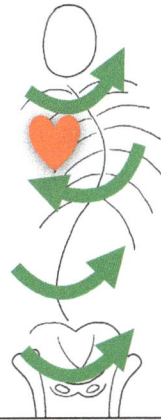

RIGHT UPPER SPINE CURVE
from the back view

Additionally, the front-to-back curves of the spine (sagittal curves) can be affected by scoliosis. Ideally, there should be three healthy natural curves of the spine from front to back:

1) The neck (cervical) slightly curves inward.
2) The upper back (thoracic) gently curves. backward
3) The lower back (lumbar) curves inward again.

Imagine these natural curves of the spine as a "spring" to absorb shock. If they are disrupted, this could cause stress in the spine. In scoliosis, these curves can become exaggerated, flattened, or even reversed in their direction.

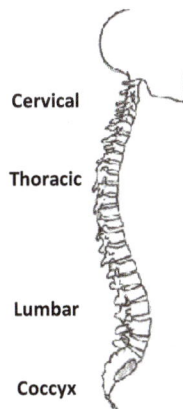

Cervical

Thoracic

Lumbar

Coccyx

There is a theory that the stress of these disrupted curves is what causes the side-to-side (lateral) curves and rotations to become worse.

This front-to-back (sagittal) set of natural curves includes the neck and it is important to note that since we all spend too much time looking down at our electronic devices, we can lose this important alignment. This loss of the cervical curve can create many neck issues, discomfort, and joint degeneration later in life. Sleeping on a good pillow with neck and head support is important as well. Also, we need to adopt a healthier posture while looking at our devices, reading, or doing computer work. I will discuss sagittal curves more along with "Text Neck" specifically in Chapters 7 and 12.

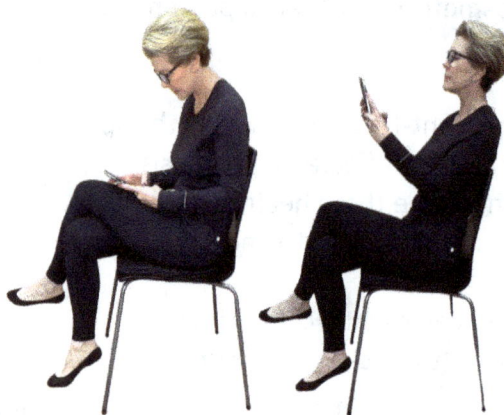

"Text Neck" Before and After Correction

What areas are affected by scoliosis?
Scoliosis is a <u>three-dimensional</u> condition that affects the:

- SHOULDER GIRDLE - it may rotate.
- SPINE - it may side bend (Single or multiple areas).
- RIB CAGE - it may rotate and displace the ribs.
- PELVIS - it may rotate and or shift side to side.
- SAGITTAL CURVES - front-to-back curves of the spine may flatten or become magnified.

See the blocks in the illustration below showing lateral curves, rotations and counter rotations to try and balance the body.

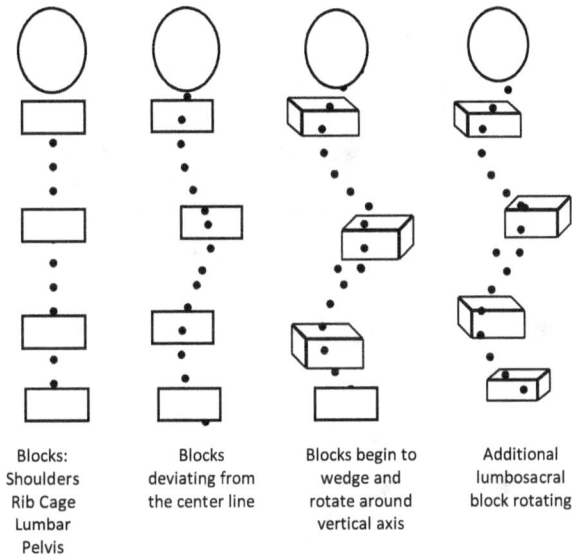

Blocks:
Shoulders
Rib Cage
Lumbar
Pelvis

Blocks
deviating from
the center line

Blocks begin to
wedge and
rotate around
vertical axis

Additional
lumbosacral
block rotating

Very severe, scoliosis can affect the heart and lungs, brain, central nervous system and the body's hormonal and digestive systems.

Famous Figures with Scoliosis:
   Yo-yo ma - musician/cellist
   Hussein (Usain) Bolt - Olympic athlete
   Sarah Michelle Gellar - actress
   Lourdes "Lola" Ciccone Leon (Madonna's daughter)
   Elizabeth Taylor - actress
   King Tut - Pharaoh of Egypt
   Alexander the Great - King of Macedon
   Liza Minnelli - actress
   Vanessa Williams - Miss America 1984/Singer/Actress
   Douglas Mac Arthur - General of the US Army
   King Richard the III of England

2. DIAGNOSING SCOLIOSIS

There are multiple ways to diagnose scoliosis.

     X-rays
     CT/CAT scan
     MRI
     Physical exam
     Scoliometer measurements
     Neurological Tests (Reflexes etc.)
     Orthopedic Tests (Physical tests)

When scoliosis is analyzed by a physician the previous tests should be used to determine the following:

Types: Structural or non-structural scoliosis (discussed later)
The Shape of the Curve: single, double, or more than 2 curves
Location: C = cervical spine, T = thoracic spine and L = lumbar spine
Direction: The convex side (outside of the curve) and whether it bends outward to the right or left.
Magnitude: The degrees of the curves are based on imaging (MRI or X-ray) measurements, called a Cobb Angle (See illustration)
Effect on Sagittal Curves: Front-to-back curves of the spine
Rotation: Each curve can cause rotation of the spine and ribs and possibly the shoulders and/or the pelvis. The degree of rotation of the spine and ribs can be measured by the use of a Scoliometer.
Causes of scoliosis: (If known)
Skeletal maturity

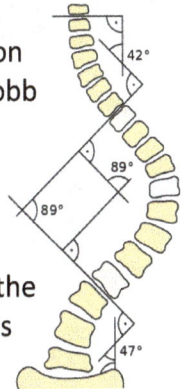

Medical terminology that you might need to know.
With scoliosis, the convex side (outward curve) is what the curve is named for. For example, it's called right scoliosis if the apex (most tilted vertebrae) bends outward to the right. Sometimes, medical terms are used instead of right or left (Dextro = Right, Levo = Left). Also, the area of the spine will be defined as thoracic (upper back), Lumbar (low back), or a combination of thoracic-lumbar. Please reference Chapter 18 "Abbreviations/Definitions/Terminology".

Let's Discuss Each of the Imaging Techniques.
X-rays are the most common tool used to diagnose and evaluate scoliosis. The scoliosis curve is measured on the image to calculate the curve in degrees ("Cobb Angle").

A child at risk of a curve worsening may be monitored periodically (usually at 3–6-month intervals) using an X-ray. The "watch and wait" method is a poor idea as a curve can progress very quickly in the first hormone surge of a child or young adult. Adults can also progress up to 1 degree per year if left untreated. This will be discussed in greater detail, later. Once a curve is measured recommendations may be made by a physician and/or the therapist. They differ as you can see in this table.

Cobb Angle / Curve Degrees	Medical Model	Schroth Therapy Model
0-20°	Observe for progression (80% of all cases).	Rather than "observation", start basic Schroth, proper posture during daily living to reduce possible curve progression.
20-25°	Brace if progressing & substantial growth is remaining.	Bracing and more aggressive postural / Schroth therapy.
25-30°	Brace if progressive and growth remains.	Studies show Schroth therapy and hard bracing creates the best results.
40-50°	Surgery is recommended in the medical community.	Studies show Schroth therapy and hard bracing creates the best results.

Types of X-rays and Other Imaging:

X-rays
EOS® X-rays
3D Ultrasound
CT/CAT Scan (Computerized tomography)
MRI (Magnetic resonance imaging)

X-ray or radiography uses a very small dose of ionizing radiation to produce pictures of the internal structures. X-rays are the oldest and most frequently used form of medical imaging.

Ways to reduce radiation:
Ask the physician to measure with a scoliometer before referring to X-ray
Reducing the number of X-rays to as few as possible
Reducing the exposed area with a smaller view (Narrow beam)
Use lead or metal shields on breasts and reproductive organs
Take an X-ray with the patient's back toward the X-ray beam
Have the patient stand at least 6 feet from the machine
Ask the radiology technician to use a filter (Called a wedge)
Ask the radiology department to use fast conventional or rare-earth films (because you don't need the highest resolution to calculate Cobb angles of scoliosis)
Use and EOS X-ray and ask for micro-dose

EOS® imaging is an X-ray technology using about 1/7th of the radiation than in traditional X-rays or CT scans. It is an ideal imaging method but it can be expensive and not available at all imaging centers. EOS can simultaneously take full-body, frontal and side-view images in a weight-bearing standing or sitting position.

A study in 2016 concluded that micro-dose EOS provided useful images of the spine while significantly reducing radiation exposure. It suggests that patients with scoliosis undergo a standard initial x-ray for full diagnosis purposes and micro-dose EOS for follow-up purposes if there is no suspicion of bone metastasis, fracture or other complaints, to reduce the accumulation of ionizing radiation in the long term.

3D Ultrasound scanning is at an early stage of development and still has some limitations.

CT / CAT Scan (computerized tomography) computers create 3-D cross-sectional images of the soft tissues, bones and blood vessels and get more detailed information than X-rays. During the minimally invasive and quick scan, the patient lies in a tunnel-like machine while the computer rotates and takes images from different angles. The doctor may use a special dye called contrast material to see structures more clearly. The patient drinks a liquid containing the contrast, or the contrast may need to be injected or given via an enema. CT/CAT Scan is less commonly used and is gradually being replaced by MRIs (Magnetic resonance imaging).

MRI (Magnetic resonance imaging)
MRIs involve no radiation as with CT/CAT scans or X-rays but they tend to be much more expensive and require the patient to hold still for long periods of time in the MRI machine which is a large machine that you lie down in. There are conditions to taking an MRI such as possible issues with metal implants, pacemakers, or magnetic devices with some types of expanding rods as we will see later in the Surgery Chapter. A new standing MRI is becoming more available and will give a more accurate picture of scoliosis since the person is not resting and relaxed but is standing in a weight-bearing position to see the natural state of the spine. An MRI is usually required by the doctor if a child is under ten years

of age, has rapidly progressing scoliosis, or has other risk factors that should be ruled out with this type of more detailed imaging.

Getting images from the medical provider.
The images will most likely be digital images that can be uploaded to a portal accessed with a password or provided to you on a CD/disc. Disc technology is becoming old and problematic. It is usually impossible for you to open the disc at home as it requires a special program. Some discs are only compatible with certain computers and are often corrupt or blank or won't open under the best conditions. If you can get your images on a portal it will be much easier to access, make a screenshot or share with other medical providers and keep them for your files. You own these images and are entitled to have access to them. Do not allow a facility to keep this information from you. Always ask that the disc be double-checked to be sure it contains the correct images and is functional before leaving the clinic.

How Often / How Should X-rays Be Taken?
(See also Chapter 9 "Bracing" for more X-ray information)

Studies suggest using X-rays on three occasions only:
- At the initial visit to confirm the diagnosis
- When there has been rapid growth or change in the curve appearance
- Before surgery to locate the exact levels for spinal fusion

Other occasions to get imaging may be to evaluate how well a brace is working during or after treatment or to monitor a scoliosis curve.

Radiation Exposure and Different Imaging Techniques
Mgy = megagray
mGy = milligray

SI = system of units of the gray (Absorption of 1 joule of radiation energy per kilogram of matter). *(Richards et al. 2010).*

The following table shows the differences in radiation doses with different types of imaging.

	Full spine film	
Imaging Techniques	**Frontal (mGy)**	**Lateral (mGy)**
EOS® microdose	0.019	0.044
EOS® low dose	0.132	0.214
Conventional X-ray	1.662	1.862
Full spine CT scan	15.6	-
Low dose full spine CT scan	5	-

How Should I Take an X-ray?
X-rays of the entire spine (including the pelvis and neck) while standing and weight-bearing are the most informative way to see the entire spine. If a full spine image is possible it is preferred but separate images may be taken and then patched together if necessary but may interfere with measuring.

It is important to take X-rays at the same time of day if they are to be taken multiple times during the growing process. At the end of the day, the curvature will seem worse than it does at the

beginning of the day due to muscle fatigue and gravity pulling on the skeleton. We are all shorter at the end of the day!
X-rays can be taken two ways:

A "back to front" (P-A view) means the back is facing the X-ray beam.

A "front to back" (A-P view) means the front is facing the X-ray beam.

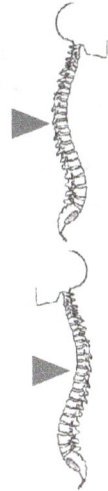

The Pros and Cons are:

- Front to back view produces better image quality.
- Back to front view substantially reduces the patient's radiation dose.

Taking an X-ray from the side (lateral or sagittal) is very important to see the posture of the "front to back" curves of the spine. To get the best possible side view, the position of the person does matter. De Sèze *et al* compared three different standing positions.

A. The clavicle position

B. The folding position

C. The straight-out arm position

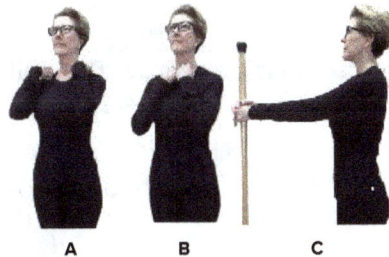

Studies found that C., the straight-out arm position, *i.e.* standing with arms and hands supported horizontally in front of the body is the closest to the natural standing posture for an X-ray.

If back pain is present, a lateral radiograph of the spine including the lumbosacral region is important to check for vertebral abnormalities such as a fracture of the spine, spondylolisthesis (a slipping forward of one vertebral bone), infection, or bony destruction of any kind. Pain may also indicate that an MRI should be taken instead of, or as well as, an X-ray.

However, a lateral X-ray should only be taken during the first series. It does not need to be taken on every follow-up X-ray unless the patient has a significant curvature.

Bracing and X-rays:
(See more information in Chapter 9 "Bracing")
It is important to do an X-ray while wearing the brace shortly after being fitted for a brace to see how much correction is being made. The side view of the correction is also very important since the front-to-back curves are just as important as the rotations and the side-to-side curves. It is critical to make sure a brace is making good corrections in all three dimensions so that any adjustments can be made to the brace.

If a patient is wearing a brace, it is not best practice to take the brace off and do an X-ray immediately. It is essential to see if the spine is holding stable after removing the brace for some time before taking an X-ray. This will allow the spine to relax into a more realistic position and reveal the correction made by the brace. Discuss how to take imaging with your brace physician and not just with the orthopedist or pediatrician.

How do X-rays Show Skeletal/Bone Maturity?
X-rays are used to measure scoliosis but also to see the status of bone development and to measure how much growth or bone maturity remains in a child. This is one important way to predict how much a scoliosis might progress. No method is perfect in predicting bone maturity, but they are all useful.

Bone maturity is measured utilizing one of several methods:

- Sanders, Greulich-Pyle, Tanner-Whitehouse and the Thumb Ossification Composite Index (TOCI) methods are based on an X-ray of the left hand and the state of ossification ("sealing" of the growth plates) of the bones.

- Risser Sign is based on an X-ray of pelvic bones which I will discuss later.

Progression of scoliosis happens mostly when bone maturity is not finished and "growth spurts" are still occurring, so intervention during this period is critical. The status of a young woman's first period (the medical term is "menarche") is also a predictor of maturity but as you can see in the research provided, these are imperfect predictors of growth, maturity, or risk of curve progression. It is important to realize that the progression of scoliosis can still happen even after bone maturity or the beginning of a girl's period.
During a" growth spurt," a curve can experience rapid worsening and it is very important to realize that "watching and waiting" even for a few weeks may be risky.

This chart tracks curve progression and the missing X-ray or exam opportunities with "watch and wait".

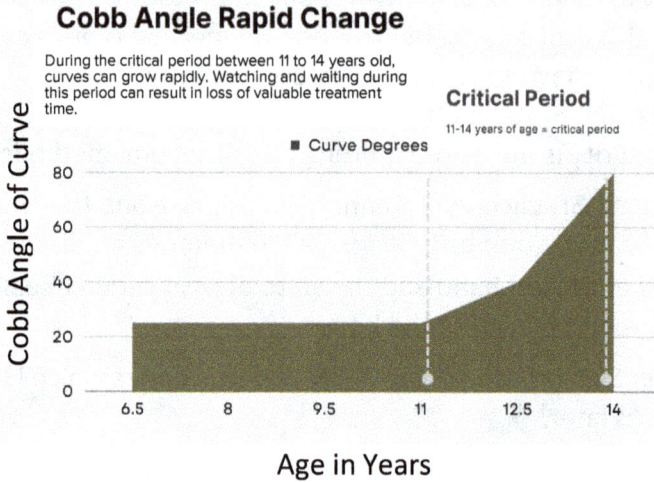

Cobb Angle Rapid Change

During the critical period between 11 to 14 years old, curves can grow rapidly. Watching and waiting during this period can result in loss of valuable treatment time.

Critical Period

11-14 years of age = critical period

■ Curve Degrees

Cobb Angle of Curve

80

60

40

20

0

6.5   8   9.5   11   12.5   14

Age in Years

If scoliosis changes rapidly with growth spurts, why don't most doctors check more frequently?

The reasons may include:

- Some doctors believe it will stabilize or resolve on its own.
- Some doctors want to avoid radiation exposure caused by repeated X-rays.
- Some doctors believe that nothing works to stop curve progression unless it has reached the "surgical range" of 40-50º in which case, a scoliosis fusion surgery is recommended.

So what can you do instead of "watch and wait"?

- Get an MRI instead of an X-ray if you or your doctor are worried about radiation

- Start scoliosis-specific postural exercise (SSPE) with a trained therapist.

- Get a highly corrective brace as soon as possible.

- Monitor growth monthly with a scoliometer for growth "spurts". This will give you a good indication of when a child is most at risk for getting worse.

What is the Risser Sign and why is it important?
When any imaging is taken of the spine it is important to include the pelvis to see the signs of bone maturity at the top of the pelvic bones. The large bones of the pelvis are called the iliac bones and the very top of the iliac bone is called the iliac crest. During the maturation process, there is a small line that is visible on imaging that shows the stages of bone maturity. This is called the Risser sign. In a child, it will appear as though there is a small hairline crack at the top of the iliac crest. This "crack" starts to fill in with solid bone during puberty from the outside rim towards the inside closest to the spine. As the line starts to fill in it is graded 0-5. Zero is the youngest and the growth spurt hasn't happened yet or has barely started, Risser 3 is when puberty is almost complete and Risser 4 or 5 is full skeletal maturity.

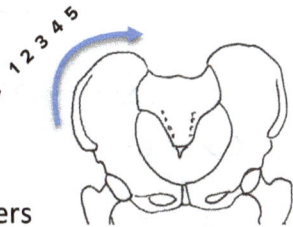

The other measuring technique is the Sanders based on an X-ray of the left hand and the state of ossification ("sealing" of the growth plates) of the bones.

Am I Done with Scoliosis Treatment at Bone Maturity?
Once bone maturity is reached at Sanders or Risser 4-5, it is more difficult to make a positive impact on the curvature in general. This is not to say in any way that people at a Risser/Sanders 4-5 should give up. Much more change can be made to the spine especially if the spine is flexible and the person is willing and motivated. Most doctors tell patients and their parents to abandon any bracing or therapy at, or near, skeletal maturity. It is important to note that there have been many cases where the curve got worse again once bracing and therapy were abandoned too soon or brace weaning was done too quickly. Studies show that bracing past the Risser 4 stage continues to have a positive impact on the curvature. You can even start bracing at a Risser 4 and have a good result. It is never too late to try.

Visual Assessment:
Scoliosis can go unnoticed in the early stages or you may begin to notice the following signs:

While standing - observe from the back:
- Observe the head - is there a tilt off to one side?
- Observe the shoulders - is one more forward?
- Observe the shoulder blades - is one more prominent on the ribcage or higher?
- Observe the ribcage - is there a prominence in the back or front?
- What happens when the person bends over at the waist? Is there a "bump" on one side?
- Observe the waist - is there a fold on one side?
- Observe the hips - one hip may seem higher or more prominent to the side than the other.

<u>From the side:</u>

- Observe the upper spine - is it flat or hyperkyphotic (Too rounded)?

- Observe the lumbar spine - is it flat or hyperlordotic (Too arched)?

<u>While lying down face up:</u>
Observe if one of the following is one more pronounced forward

- Shoulders

- Ribs

- Hips

As seen in Chapter 1 "What is Scoliosis", another way to understand what is happening in the body is: Imagine "blocks" that distort during scoliosis. Observe the blocks below. Imagine the larger part of the block as moving backwards, meaning; that area is leaning outward laterally into the wide block AND rotating backward. The small part of the wedge is leaning inward laterally AND rotating forward.

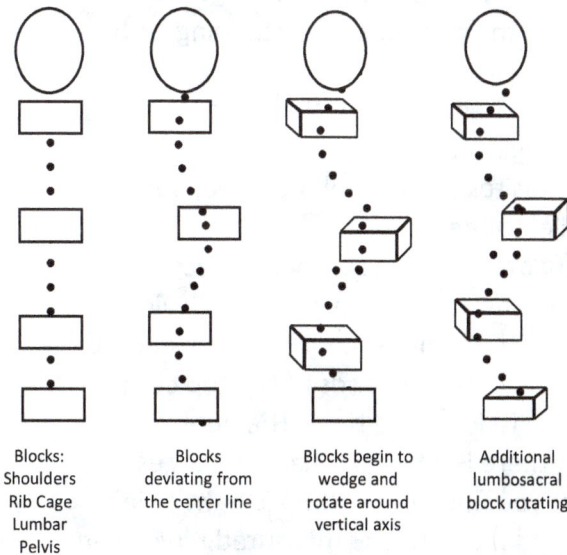

| Blocks: Shoulders Rib Cage Lumbar Pelvis | Blocks deviating from the center line | Blocks begin to wedge and rotate around vertical axis | Additional lumbosacral block rotating |

If any of these signs are noted, it is wise to get evaluated as soon as possible. If the individual is still growing, scoliosis can progress very quickly in childhood and even in the late teen years.

The Adam's Test: (see Chapter 20, page 231 "Scoliosis Screening Handout") Scoliosis shows its telltale "bump" in a forward-bend position. A Scoliometer device can measure the locations and degrees of spinal rotations that cause the "bump". Usually, this test is performed in school but is being given less frequently in the US. Ask a pediatrician or school nurse to perform the test or purchase a scoliometer for home use. It is simple to learn how to use and online videos are available. Visit my Scoliosis Coach YouTube Channel: https://youtu.be/-I4JH-3aaJc To purchase a scoliometer, visit my website www.ScoliosisCoach.com

How to Perform the Adams Test and Use a Scoliometer:

Wearing a sports bra, or otherwise exposed back and no shoes, stand with feet together.
1. Sit behind the person who is standing with their back to you.
2. The person bends over at the waist with straight legs and straight and relaxed arms with palms together, until the upper spine is parallel to the floor.
3. Upper back: Place the scoliometer across the back with the "cut out" part of the device straddling the bony center of the spine. Hold the device with two hands at the top corners and move it down the back. The bubble will move if there is a bump. Chart the largest number you find, if the bump is right or left, where and the date you measured it (you can

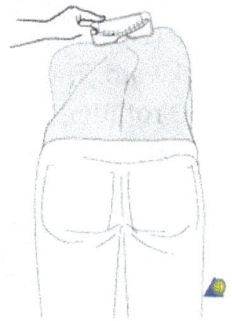

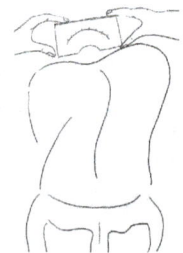

RIGHT UPPER SPINE
CURVE (from the back)

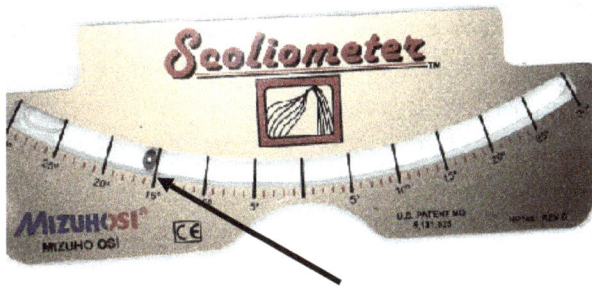

use stickers on the side of the spine if you wish to mark the rotations). I provide a Scoliosis Screening Chart at the end of this handbook.

4. Lower back: As you approach the low back the person may need to bend further over until the lumbar spine is parallel to the floor. Continue moving to the lowest part of the back.

Mark the largest number, if the bump is Right or Left, where and the date you measured it.

Do not press down hard on the scoliometer device. That can distort the reading. Retest again 1-2 times for accuracy. Keep a journal or use the Scoliosis Screening Chart mentioned earlier.

What do the numbers mean? As seen in the photo above, the bubble goes to one side, meaning the opposite side was the higher side or the rotated area. This image indicates a 16º rotation of the right, the higher side.

In a patient, when 5° of rotation or more is seen, or a significant increase in degrees over some time, a physician should evaluate it, especially if you are testing a person who is still growing.

For more details on how a doctor should screen for scoliosis and diagnose it, see Chapter 14 "Choosing a Doctor".

_Note__: Remember, true scoliosis is not only side-to-side curvature but also has a rotational element. A scoliotic curve _<u>_without rotation_</u>_ should be investigated for other causes, including bony tumors, neuromuscular conditions, intraspinal pathology and nerve root irritation._

3. TYPES OF SCOLIOSIS

The type of scoliosis is partly determined by the patient's age at the time of diagnosis.

Type of Scoliosis by Age:
Infantile idiopathic (unknown origin) scoliosis (IIS):
Diagnosed between birth and 3+ (before four years).

Early onset scoliosis (EOS): *Not to be confused with EOS X-ray!*
Diagnosed between birth and ten years.

Juvenile idiopathic scoliosis (JIS):
Diagnosed between four and ten years.

Adolescent idiopathic scoliosis (AIS):
Diagnosed between ten and eighteen years.

Patients with IIS and JIS are grouped under the EOS umbrella. EOS can be caused by an underlying condition or have no known cause.

There are Two Main Types of Scoliosis:
Structural and Non-Structural and it can be confusing. There is a big difference between structural and nonstructural scoliosis.

Nonstructural Scoliosis is also called functional Scoliosis. Nonstructural scoliosis is less serious and tends not to alter the body structurally. This type of curve disappears when an image is taken lying down or bending sideways. It can be caused by a variety of reasons including muscle spasms, leg length discrepancy, injury, poor posture, or repeated unbalanced activities such as carrying heavy loads long term on one side.

Nonstructural scoliosis tends to have only a small degree of curvature and therefore is usually much less noticeable. It is almost always reversible.

Structural Scoliosis means a spinal curvature that is always present. It is evident in imaging taken standing, lying on the back, or bending sideways and is considered permanent unless the spine receives treatment such as exercise, scoliosis-specific postural exercises (SSPE), bracing, or surgery. An easy test for structural scoliosis is the forward bending test also called the Adams Test as I previously discussed.

This book focuses on idiopathic/structural scoliosis since it is the most common type. It involves a side-to-side curvature as well as spinal rotations. See below.

Types of Structural Scoliosis

•**Idiopathic scoliosis** means the cause is unknown. This type usually develops during the onset of puberty/adolescence and is called "AIS" (meaning adolescent idiopathic scoliosis), but it can start earlier. Idiopathic scoliosis is by far the most common and the only type that will be covered in this book.

- 80-90% of scoliosis cases fall into this category.

- 80% is found in girls and girls' curves progress more often than boys.

- It is usually evident in girls between 10 and 14 years of age and boys between 12 and 15 years.

- 80% is on the right side of the upper spine.

- During puberty, the spine is more pliable and intervention can reduce the curve substantially.

- Most cases are very slight curvatures under 20° Cobb angle on imaging.

• If left untreated, the curve can worsen quickly during puberty.

Other causes of scoliosis which are not classified as idiopathic are.....

• **Degenerative scoliosis** is also known as adult-onset scoliosis, late-onset scoliosis, or de novo scoliosis and is often linked to loss of bone or disc health. The structures of the spine can degenerate due to osteoporosis or arthritis and cause a bone or bones, to "wedge shape" and lead to a curvature of the spine.

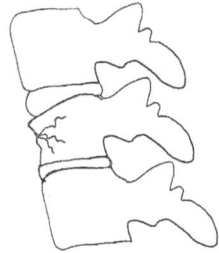

• **Congenital scoliosis** is a rare condition (1 in 10,000) that develops before birth. These cases are usually benign and often require no treatment.

Formation Defects: a malformation in the vertebrae of the spine that may be asymmetric or incorrectly shaped, for example, a half vertebra called a wedge or hemivertebrae. In some cases, it may be corrected surgically. It usually becomes apparent at the age of two years when the spine is growing quickly and it puts extra strain on the abnormal bones.

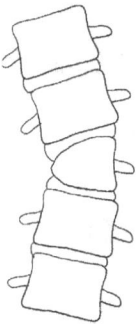

Segmentation Defects: (one-sided bar formation, rib synostosis) when ribs fuse or a bar of bone joins two bones together. These conditions commonly are combined.

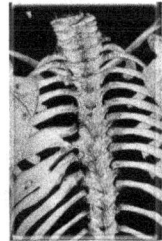

• **Osteochondrodysplasia** is a general term for rare genetic disorders of bone development causing generalized skeletal functional issues. An MRI is usually needed to get a more detailed diagnosis of the type.

•**Scheuermann's Disease** (Juvenile kyphosis) is a rounding of the spine backward and usually affects the upper back. Scheuermann's kyphosis is diagnosed or appears at 12-13 years old during adolescence. It affects males more commonly (Ratio is 2:1 for males, of unknown cause). It develops as a result of some structural deformity in the bones of the spine. Wedging of the vertebrae of 5º or more (front to back) can occur over 3 adjacent vertebrae = Scheuermann's diagnosis. Also associated are irregular end-plates of the vertebral bodies and Schmorl's nodes (invagination of the disc into the bodies of the vertebrae). This can occur in the lumbar spine too and cause a reversed or flat lordosis). Early symptoms remain fairly consistent and they generally do not worsen over time except in severe cases and include: poor posture ("hunched over"), back pain, muscle fatigue and stiffness in the back.

•**Neuromuscular scoliosis** is the second most frequent type of scoliosis after idiopathic and is caused when the brain and muscles are unable to communicate well. It is likely that the curve will progress and can become severe. Almost all children will require surgery at some point. However, sometimes braces are used to slow the curve's progression until a later time when surgery can be safely performed. Kyphosis is also frequently present. There are two types, neuropathic (nerves) and myopathic (muscular) and include conditions such as cerebral palsy, spinal cord trauma, tethered cord, Chiari malformation, neurofibromatosis, Marfan syndrome, Ehlers-Danlos, Prader-Willi and muscular dystrophy. *VIP: A scoliotic curve without rotation should be screened for other causes, including neuromuscular conditions, bony tumors and nerve root irritation explained below.*

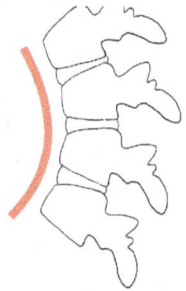

Let's explore a few of these neuromuscular conditions further.

Tethered cord syndrome:
(also called fastened cord
syndrome) is a condition
in which the spinal cord is
stuck, or fixed inside the
spinal canal. This causes
tightness of the spinal
cord as a child grows. This
tight spinal cord results in

Normal Brain / Chiari I Malformation

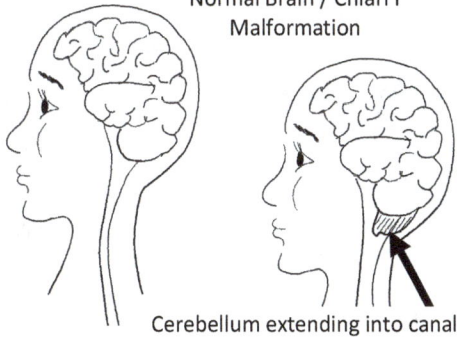

Cerebellum extending into canal

a tugging force on the bones of the spinal column, causing the
column to compress down and bend into scoliosis in response to
the nerve tension. Symptoms include
back pain or shooting pain in the legs, Normal Spinal Nerves / Tethered Nerves
weakness, numbness or problems
with muscle function in the legs
including shaking or spasms, changes
in the feet: higher arches or curled
toes, repeated bladder infections,
loss of bladder or bowel control that
gets worse, scoliosis that changes or
gets worse, seen on the back: a fatty
mass, dimple, birthmark or a tuft of
hair. Incidentally, there are Schroth exercise protocols for this
condition.

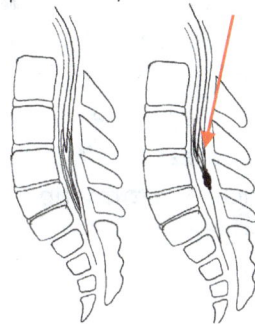

Chiari Malformation: There are a few types of Chiari
Malformations

• Chiari I Malformation is most common. Parts of the lower brain
hang down through the opening in the base of the skull into the
upper neck. Most often, this happens while a baby is developing
in the womb because the back of a baby's skull is too small. The

35

condition may be so mild that it does not cause symptoms until later in life. 20% of these patients have scoliosis.

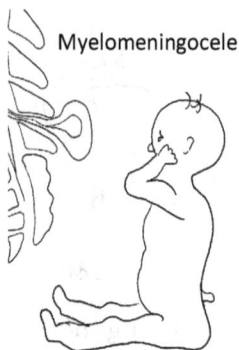
Myelomeningocele

• Chiari II Malformation: The bottom of the brain and parts of the brainstem hangs down into the neck. This type also develops before birth. Children with this type also have a serious form of spina bifida called myelomeningocele. This is a defect when the baby's spine, the spinal cord and the spinal canal do not form or close normally.

Syringomyelia/Syrinx is a disorder in which a fluid-filled cyst (called a syrinx) forms within the spinal cord. Over time, the cyst/syrinx can get bigger and may damage the spinal cord and compress and injure the nerve fibers. Chiari Malformation is combined with syringomyelia up to 50-60% of the time. Scoliosis appears in 50% of these cases.

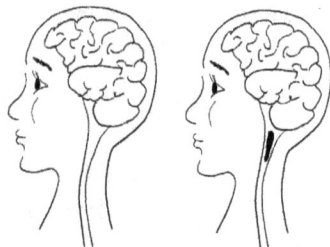
Normal Brain / Syrinx in Cord

An orthopedic test to check for these neuromuscular conditions is called the Cox Test which checks for nervous system tension (the same test done for disc problems and sciatica). The patient is lying down with the upper back and head propped up at a sharp angle and a bolster under the neck and low back to create tension in the

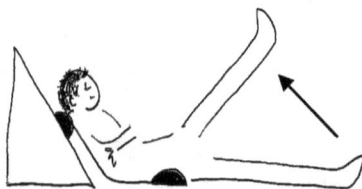

spinal cord. The legs are straight as one leg is slowly lifted by the physician to see if the hip suddenly lifts which can indicate increased nervous system tension that should be further evaluated.

Curve Classification: will be covered in Chapter 9 "Bracing".

Most Common Scoliosis Presentations:

- Thoracic (upper back): 90% of thoracic scoliosis curves outward to the right. This is usually associated with a rib bump on the right side of the upper back.

- Lumbar (lower back): 65 to 70% of lumbar scoliosis curves outwards to the left.

- Thoracolumbar: curve can capture both the upper and lower back (80% curve to the right).

- Double S or S-shaped curvature is the combination of two curves: upper and lower spine in opposite directions of each other providing a possible counterbalance. Prognosis is best when the curves are symmetrical.

4. CAUSES OF SCOLIOSIS

Studies have ruled out the idea that adolescent idiopathic scoliosis curves are caused by specific behaviors such as regularly carrying heavy loads or "bad posture", but that does not mean that these don't have any impact on scoliosis. Posture correction and knowing what to avoid do matter and will be covered in Chapter 11 "What Should I Avoid?" and Chapter 12 "Exercise and Scoliosis"

The different types of scoliosis have already been outlined.

- Structural (Idiopathic, degenerative, congenital, neuromuscular)
- Non-Structural (Muscle spasm, leg length, injury)

Some of those types have a clear explanation of what caused scoliosis. Although idiopathic scoliosis is the most common type and is defined as having no known cause, research and technology are being improved all the time to find a possible cause.

Genetics

Scoliosis appears to involve genetic hereditary factors because it sometimes runs in families. Adults with idiopathic scoliosis should have their children carefully screened. Studies have shown: Siblings are 7 times more likely to have scoliosis if one child has it. Children are 3 times more likely to have scoliosis if a parent has it.

Genetic factors influencing the progression of adolescent idiopathic scoliotic curves are still being analyzed with DNA samples from blood and saliva. There is a pretty wide medical acceptance that genetic factors do play a role but this is still being studied as of the date of publication.

In 2010 a company named Axial Biotech released the first genetic DNA saliva test called the ScoliScore test for predicting if scoliosis in a teenager would likely get worse. Unfortunately, three separate independent researchers were unable to reproduce the findings of the initial study.

Research is underway on the following issues:

- DNA
- Hormones
- Low melatonin - signaling pathway disruption possibly influencing growth mechanisms
- Vit D
- CA
- Magnesium
- Biomechanics
- Leptin

5. HORMONES AND SCOLIOSIS

In the course of life, we have normal hormonal fluctuations and these fluctuations may affect scoliosis, so it is best to be aware of them.

What fluctuations?

- Growth Spurt #1: Growth spurt 0-6 years

- Growth Spurt #2: Puberty and first growth hormone surge approx. 12 years to skeletal maturity. This is the **most important time to diagnose and treat scoliosis early**. This table outlines when the growth spurts occur.

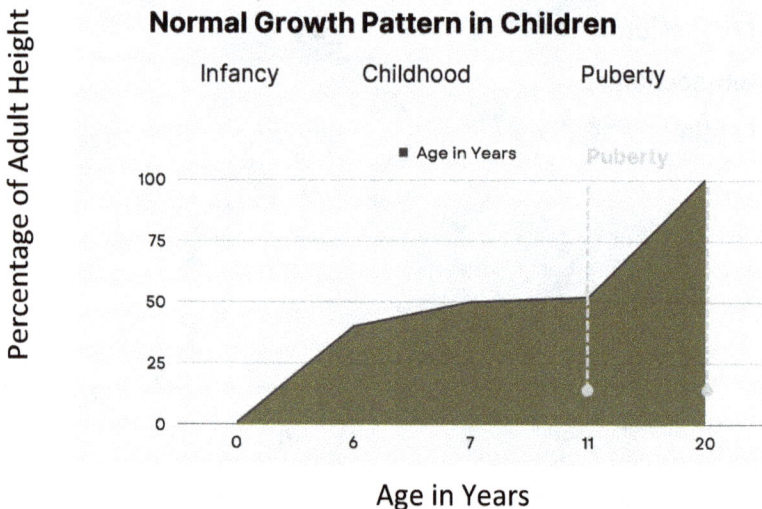

Normal Growth Pattern in Children

Infancy   Childhood   Puberty

Percentage of Adult Height

- Age in Years

Puberty

100

75

50

25

0

0   6   7   11   20

Age in Years

- Pregnancy / Fertility Treatment: During pregnancy and fertility treatment, Relaxin hormone is produced in the body to relax the ligaments to facilitate childbirth. An existing scoliosis curve can worsen at this time due to the laxity of the ligaments throughout the body including the spine.

- Menopause: The drop of estrogen in female menopause causes bone loss which can lead to a worsening of existing scoliosis. Women on HRT (hormone replacement therapy) have been shown to have LESS curve progression than those who do not go on HRT.

- Some diseases that disturb hormones and can affect bone density are:

- Primary hyperparathyroidism

- Hyperthyroidism

- Hypogonadism

- Growth hormone deficiency

- Cushing's syndrome

- Anorexia nervosa

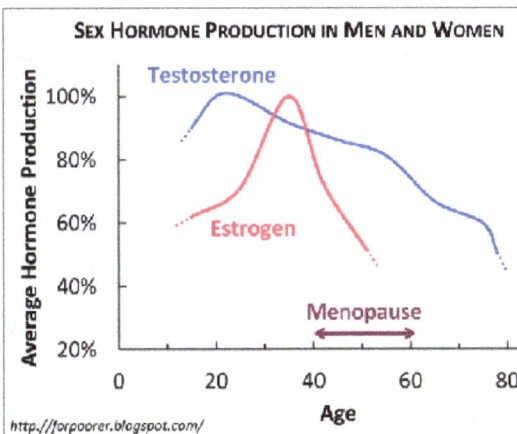

SEX HORMONE PRODUCTION IN MEN AND WOMEN

http://forpoorer.blogspot.com/

These conditions frequently cause secondary osteoporosis which could lead to scoliosis or a worsening of existing scoliosis. Certain medications and drugs can pull minerals from bones and lead to osteoporosis as well. Always consult with your doctor about medication concerns, side effects, or interactions with other drugs.

- Anticoagulants (Heparin, Warfarin)
- Anti-epileptic drugs
- Steroid drugs (Oral or inhaled)
- High doses of thyroid medicines
- Certain diabetes medicines
- Certain cancer drugs
- Certain stomach medicines (Antacids containing aluminum)
- Certain antidepressants
- Progestins (A hormone in many forms of contraception and hormone replacement products)
- Nicotine
- Alcohol
- Street drugs such as methamphetamine, cocaine and opioids
- Where these factors are present, be careful to monitor curves closely and be proactive in exercise or support of the spine.

This table outlines when a curve can grow rapidly according to age.

Cobb Angle Rapid Change

During the critical period between 11 to 14 years old, curves can grow rapidly. Watching and waiting during this period can result in loss of valuable treatment time.

Critical Period

11-14 years of age = critical period

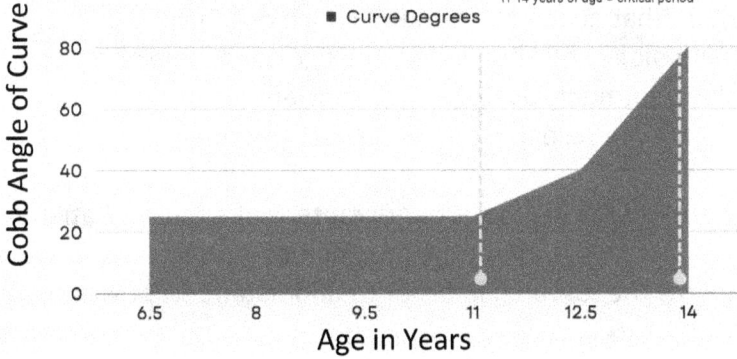

■ Curve Degrees

Cobb Angle of Curve

| 80 |
| 60 |
| 40 |
| 20 |
| 0 |

6.5   8   9.5   11   12.5   14

Age in Years

6. ALTERNATIVE SCOLIOSIS TREATMENTS & THE SCHROTH TECHNIQUE

History shows us how long we have been striving to overcome scoliosis and how many notable figures had some type of condition that needed treatment, which only helped push forward our technology and knowledge. Let's go over some of the most popular treatments available from ancient history to today and investigate the research on the newest treatments.

Be aware of false promises or guarantees of a "cure". Patients need to be realistic about the possibilities with scoliosis treatment and follow the research in order to understand what works.

Non-surgical treatment of scoliosis dates back to ancient times. King Tut and Alexander the Great most likely had scoliosis.

c. 3200 B.C.E.
Ancient Indian texts tell the story of Kubja, a maid described as having a severe deformity of her spine. Legend is that Krishna healed her by pressing on her feet while lifting her head. This is a possible description of how the ancients tried to heal scoliosis.

1524 B.C.E.
Ahmose Meritamun was an Egyptian princess and her mummy is the oldest to have been found with scoliosis.

1341 B.C.E. King Tut (Tutankhamun) likely had scoliosis as he was buried with 130 walking sticks or crutches and a special headrest possibly designed to keep his back straight. Some paintings show him using these sticks and leaning or standing strangely with his legs crossed awkwardly.

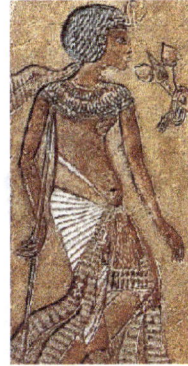

460-370 B.C.E. Hippocrates (the father of medicine) was the first to use the word scoliosis from the Greek word crooked. He invented devices called:

- The Hippocratic Ladder
- The Hippocratic board
- The Luxation table
- The Hippocratic scamnum (A rack).

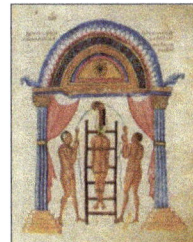

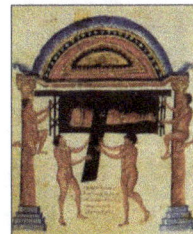

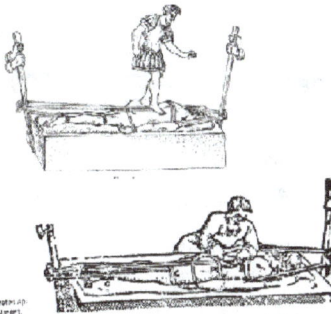

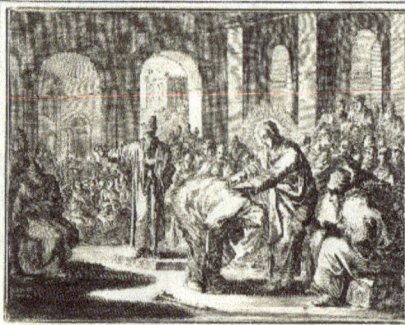

Jan Luyken, Jesus Heals the Bent Woman in the Synagogue. Dutch, 1712 Amsterdam, Rijksmuseum

20 C.E. According to the Bible (Luke 13: 10-17), Jesus performed a miracle on a stooped-over woman who likely had scoliosis.

200 C.E. A Roman named Galen expanded on Hippocrates' work by dividing spine disorders into categories with scoliosis being a specific type. This system is much the same today. He also modified Hippocrates' contraptions for treatment.

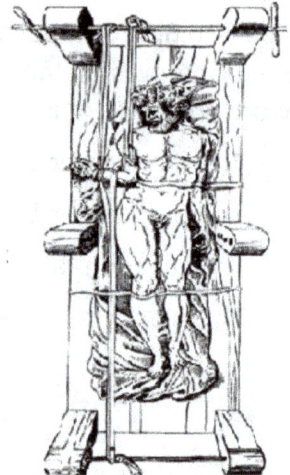

The Machine of Hippocrates (Husbert, 1967) Moe's textbook of scoliosis and other spine deformities Lonstein, J., Bradford, D., Winter, R., Ogilvie, J. (1995)

1452 C.E. King Richard III of England had scoliosis based on an examination of his skeleton found in 2013. He may have been treated with devices modified from medieval torture devices such as "the rack" created to pull the body apart in an attempt to traction the back.

1510 Ambroise Pare a French doctor, invented iron corsets for children to act as scoliosis braces to correct curves.

1820 Lewis Albert Sayre, called the founding father of orthopedics, designed the Sayre Jacket so that he could suspend and traction patients while plaster of Paris was applied to create a custom-casted scoliosis brace.

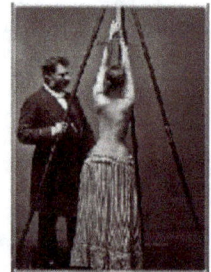

Lewis Albert Sayre and patient

46

1894 Katharina Schroth developed the Schroth Method of exercise and breathing techniques to reduce scoliosis and was the founder of exercise-based treatment.

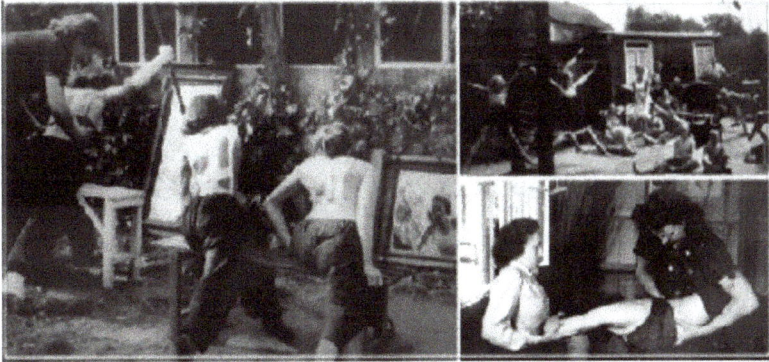

All historical photos from the picture database of ®Christa Lehnert-Schroth

1865 Dr. Paul Harrington designed the Harrington rod which was the first surgical implant to straighten the spine as the gold standard of scoliosis surgical care from the 1960s to the late 1990s.

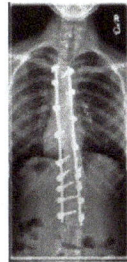

Various techniques and devices were used throughout history. Many of these general concepts still exist in treatment today in terms of traction, exercise and bracing which are all covered in our other chapters.

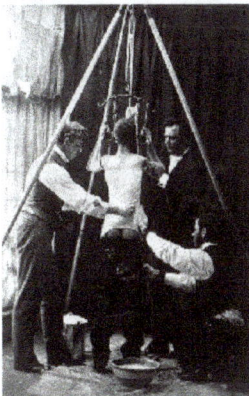

Traction with plaster casting

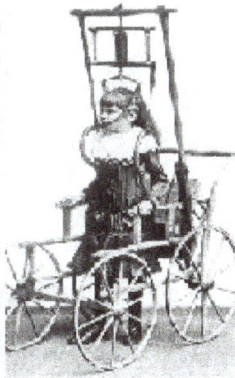

Traction carriage

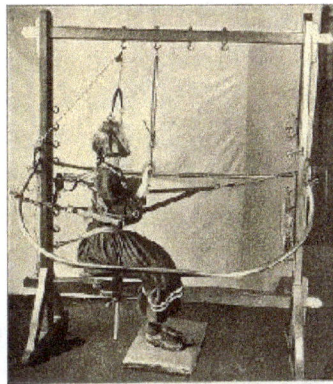

Seated traction device

I will outline each alternative treatment option:

- Chiropractic care
- Yoga/Pilates
- Acupuncture
- Massage
- Scoliosis Specific Postural Exercises (SSPE) or Physiotherapeutic Scoliosis Specific Exercises (PPSE)

Chiropractic Care

Chiropractic management of scoliosis may include manual or mechanical spinal adjustments and is sometimes combined with exercise and postural education, foot orthotics or heel lifts, electrical muscle stimulation, massage, or traction.

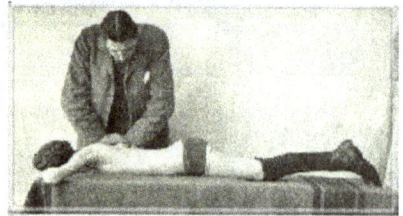

Chiropractic on scoliosis 1904

Virtually no formal research exists documenting chiropractic in managing scoliosis. Several well-conducted case studies suggest that chiropractic is, indeed, effective in managing scoliotic curves, but definitive studies are lacking. It is widely stated that chiropractic care is effective in alleviating the pain and discomfort associated with adult scoliosis. However, no studies to date have adequately documented this effect.

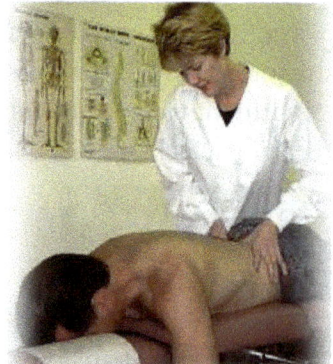

Although available evidence suggests that spinal manipulation does not halt or reverse the progression of adolescent scoliosis, it

48

may influence curve degrees on X-ray but this could be temporary and effective only in patients that are not at risk of significant progression. A Med-line search of the research did not show any evidence to suggest that chiropractic adjustments alone can be beneficial in reducing curvatures in cases of structural idiopathic scoliosis, but there is evidence to suggest that certain types of chiropractic care could improve functional scoliosis. Patients should be referred to a spinal orthopedist or neurosurgeon if the scoliosis curves keep increasing.

Yoga
There are many types and styles of yoga, from meditative to very strenuous. Although yoga has not demonstrated any scientific value in treating scoliosis, many with scoliosis say that they have felt much better when they practice yoga. This may be due to the stretching and strengthening of muscles but may not be a viable solution long-term. Why? Many of the movements in most types of yoga could be counterproductive to scoliosis in terms of rotation when there are already areas of rotation with scoliosis, flexion when the spine might already be too flexed, or extension when the spine might already be too flat and in too much extension. It is very important to understand your scoliosis fully and completely before embarking on an exercise routine that could negatively influence the curves in any way. At the same time, it is very important to create flexibility, particularly in the hips. Many yoga postures stretch the hamstrings, hip flexors and quadriceps which are the key muscles that not only create more mobility and strength but which can help improve posture. Many yoga postures also loosen the upper back, particularly the trapezius muscles. The practice of yoga also emphasizes breath awareness. With scoliosis, there is often a decreased breathing capacity on the inside of the curve (concave side) because the ribs may be compressed together and the muscles along the spine and in between the ribs lose some of their elasticity and strength.

Breathing into the compressed ribcage on the concave side creates more lung capacity and oxygenates the body, lengthens the spine, de-rotates the ribcage, strengthens the muscles on this weaker side, creates more evenness of the sides of the body and relieves pain. This directional asymmetrical breath can correct or prevent further progression of the curvature and is a critical part of a therapeutic program. Even if it is as simple as adding a deep breath during the workday or commute, breathing into the concave areas is very impactful.

If correct breathing is neglected, the breathing may automatically default into the convex/larger area and the curve can get worse over time.

Always work with an experienced instructor and know how to modify your practice for your scoliosis.

Pilates

As with yoga, Pilates may come with its list of issues. Many of the movements in Pilates may be asymmetrical or encourage rotation, extension, or flexion in areas of the spine that do not need this encouragement. It is always important to work with an experienced instructor who is knowledgeable about scoliosis and knows how to modify the practice for each particular scoliosis. At the very least you should understand your curve and how to modify your practice by learning from a trained scoliosis-specific postural exercise (SSPE) professional. The benefits of Pilates include but are not limited to posture, core strength, breath and elongation work. Joseph H. Pilates was born only 12 years before Katarina Schroth in 1883 in Mönchengladbach, Germany and was sickly

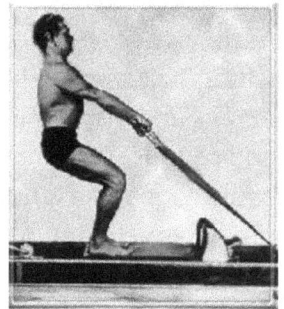

himself and went on to find his own remedies much like Schroth. It is interesting to note that these two German-born exercise pioneers lived and worked in the same era and both of them were so far ahead of their time that their methods are still used worldwide.

Acupuncture

Acupuncture uses fine needles that are intended to stimulate points in the body aimed at creating an energy flow to treat many illnesses. Recently, some reports have suggested that using acupuncture for scoliosis could improve the curve and the associated pain. For now, there is no scientific evidence that proves that its use helps in the treatment of scoliosis other than relief from pain and stress.

Massage

- Increases blood flow to the muscles and tissues
- Stretches tight areas of the body
- Relieves pain
- Enhances mobility
- Promotes better sleep

Manual therapy for scoliosis includes massage therapy and physical manipulation techniques, such as chiropractic manipulation and spinal traction. Massage therapists sometimes use multiple techniques in the treatment of scoliosis, including:

- Swedish massage: One of the most common types of massage, involves kneading, tapping, long strokes and shaking motions.
- Deep tissue massage: Stretching, deep tissue work and neuromuscular therapy to increase the flow of blood to muscles and tissues and lengthen tightened areas.

- Myofascial release: Focuses on opening up stiff areas in the tough membranes that wrap around and support the muscles.

- Cranial-sacral therapy: Helps to balance the spine and improve a person's overall function by mobilizing restricted tissue within and around the spine.

- Thai yoga massage (Thai massage) is a dynamic bodywork therapy based upon yoga and ayurveda that is done fully clothed.

Does Scoliosis Massage Work?
Only a small number of clinical studies have looked at the benefits of massage for adolescent idiopathic scoliosis. Most of these involved one or a few cases, so the results should be viewed with some caution.

Never allow a massage therapist to perform skeletal adjustments unless he or she is trained to do so.

Scoliosis Specific Postural Exercises (SSPE) or Physiotherapeutic Scoliosis Specific Exercises (PPSE)
The principle behind exercise rehabilitation programs for scoliosis is postural reeducation to reduce asymmetric spinal loading during and after growth.

The programs are designed for each patient after a clinical classification and imaging evaluation of the curvature type has been made by a doctor or therapist. It usually involves patient education, learning auto-correction in three dimensions, stabilizing the posture, training in activities of daily life (ADLs), self-elongation and specific exercises. Scoliosis-specific exercises are increasingly used in conjunction with bracing in the treatment of progressive idiopathic scoliosis and the research shows this to be the best program to effect real change.

Types of Scoliosis Specific Postural Exercises (SSPE) or Physiotherapeutic Scoliosis Specific Exercises (PPSE) include programs like:

- Scientific Exercise Approach to Scoliosis from Italy (SEAS)
- The SEAS method is an individualized exercise program adapted for medium-degree scoliosis.
- Lyon Method from France
- The Lyon method includes bracing, patient education, awareness of posture, mobilization, neuromuscular control of the spine, coordination, trunk stabilization, muscular strength, respiration and ergonomics.
- Schroth Method from Germany (Best Practice® and Asklepios)
- The Schroth Method is a nonsurgical option for scoliosis treatment. It uses exercises customized for each patient to return the curved spine to a more natural position. The goal of Schroth exercises is to de-rotate, elongate and stabilize the spine in a three-dimensional plane.
- Barcelona Scoliosis Physical Therapy School (BSPTS)
- The BSPTS-Concept by Rigo. Based on four general principles: Three-dimensional stable postural correction; Expansion Technique; Muscle activation and Integration.
- Dobomed from Poland
- The Dobomed system aims to reconstruct the physiological curve. In most cases, breath training is carried out when the patient is on the all-four position. In such a position with respiration training, the flatness of the thoracic section is adjusted and the curvature in the lumbar area is corrected.
- Functional Individual Therapy of Scoliosis from Poland (FITS)

- FITS was established in 2004 for the treatment of children, adolescents and adults with scoliosis, postural defects and Scheuermann's disease.
- Side Shift from England
- Dr. Min Mehta of England brought up Side shift treatment in 1985, which was used in Royal National Orthopaedic Hospital. This treatment relies on the movement of the body's trunk toward the concave side to achieve correction of scoliosis.

Some of the following methods use SSPE and may also include movement therapy or balancing and/or weighted devices, traction and manual manipulation. These are usually intensive programs that may involve a "boot camp" experience with intensive weekends of exercise with a take-home plan, a device to use at home and a brace that is usually elastic. These programs tend to be very expensive and the soft braces do not have good research outcomes in general.

- ScoliSMART® - utilizes specialized exercises based on Schroth principles, wearing a weighted device designed to push the curves and activate muscles, an elastic brace called the Activity Suit, the use of the Traction Chair and chiropractic manipulations.

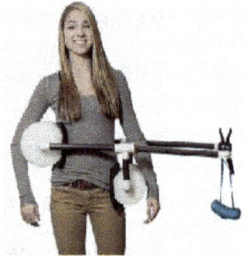

- Scolio-Fit® / NuSchroth®: utilizes specialized exercises based on Schroth, an elastic brace called the SpineCor® and chiropractic manipulations.

Studies indicate that hard bracing (with varied results based on the type of brace) and scoliosis-specific postural exercise (SSPE) performed with a therapist have a pivotal role in slowing the progression of scoliosis and reducing the size of the curve.

Importantly, SSPE reduces the loss of the correction that was achieved in a brace. Frequently when weaning off of a brace some curve correction can be lost, so continued scoliosis-specific postural exercise is vital! Important studies about what works can be found in Chapter 21 "Research".

Always be wary of any practitioner who tells you that he or she can "cure" scoliosis, as it simply is not true. Clients need to be realistic about the possibilities with scoliosis and follow the research of what works. Use these SSPE techniques to improve posture and well-being, relieve pain and help urge you along your journey to improve scoliosis in conjunction with proven therapies such as bracing under the care of certified and trained professionals.

Most of my patients have reported substantial pain relief with simple changes to their activities of daily living and postural correction even before they start doing the Schroth exercises. Interestingly, there have been cases when my patients have an emotional or physical response to exercise or are being placed into a new position either with exercise or a new posture. Feelings of being unwell and dizzy, or nauseous have happened and are usually very temporary and we just slow down and take a break before continuing. Either the position is wrong for them or it is just a reaction to breaking the scoliosis pattern that is embedded in the body, mind and spirit. If this happens to you, stop, rest, or talk with your therapist about changing it up.

The disadvantages of scoliosis therapy programs are:
- Limited access to skilled scoliosis therapists
- Lack of compliance with a home program
- A poor understanding of the home program
- Time management

- A lack of insurance coverage
- Cost

Always practice scoliosis exercises only if they were prescribed to you by a professional. One size does not fit all and the exercises must be tailored to each curve type. For a trained therapist please see Chapter 17 "Resources".

What is the Schroth Technique?
Considered the very first Scoliosis Specific Postural Exercise (SSPE) technique, Schroth is a series of exercise and breathing techniques to correct scoliosis. The method has been copied, modified and added onto by many since its creation. A Schroth therapist must be certified in the method to apply it to a patient.

The Schroth Method includes:
1) Activation and lengthening of muscles in the <u>concavities</u> of the spine
2) Correction of vertebral rotation using breathing that causes the ribs to work as levers to de-rotate the spine and improve pulmonary function
3) Elongation of the spine
4) Restoration of the sagittal curves (Front to back curves)
5) Activities of daily living to improve posture all the time, not just during the exercises.

The History of Schroth Involves the work of three generations: Katharina Schroth, Christa Lehnert-Schroth and Hans R. Weiss (Son of Christa). Katharina Schroth, born in Dresden Germany, suffered from scoliosis and was treated with a steel brace at 16 years old. She later decided to develop a treatment for herself. Katharina tried to "breathe away her deformities" by inflating the concavities and overcorrecting the curves with

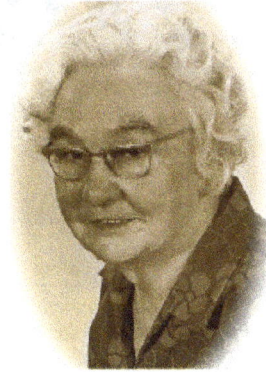

All historical photos are from the picture database of ®Christa Lehnert-Schroth

Katharina Schroth 1894-1985

specific corrective movements. These methods were published as early as 1924. She was not a professional trainer or a doctor, but she started her program as a schoolteacher who worked with gymnasts.

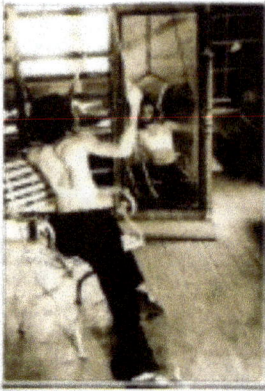

Patient with large curvature exercising in front of a mirror for monitoring and feedback.

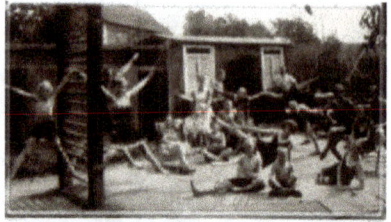

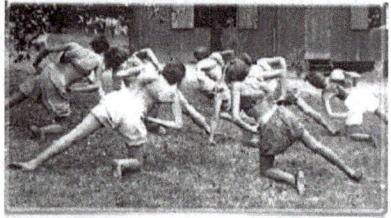

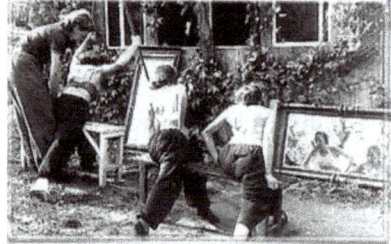

Large curvatures treated in Schroth's institute in the 30's in Meissen, Germany. Patients with curvatures exceeding 80° with huge rib humps and stiff deformities were the main focus of work.

In the 30's in Meissen, Germany, groups of patients with large curvatures exercising in the garden of the institute in front of mirrors to allow monitoring and feedback. Most of the treatment was done outside for fresh air and sunshine, at a time when people were not used to exposing their skin to the sun or to other people.

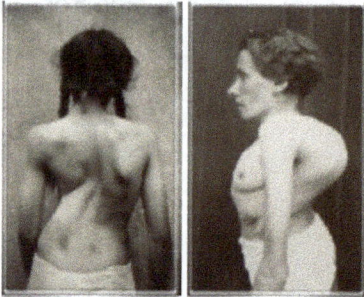

The Next Generation of Schroth

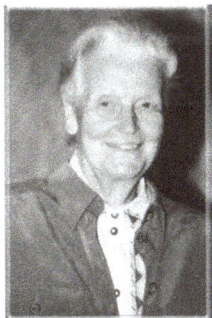

Christa Lehnert-Schroth
1924-2015

Christa Lehnert-Schroth, P.T., helped her mother, Katharina, in her clinic in Meissen (Then East Germany). In 1955, they moved to West Germany to open a new institute in Bad Sobernheim, which grew to treat up to 150 patients at a time. Christa became its director, serving until her retirement in 1995. After her divorce from Ernst Weiss, Christa Schroth married Adalbert Lehnert, who helped her in the clinic and the treatment of patients.

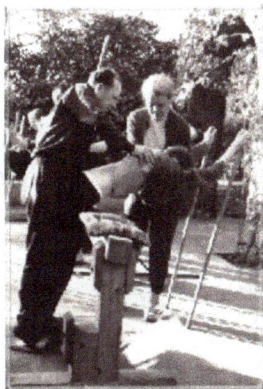

She trained hundreds of therapists in the Schroth method and supervised the treatment of more than 10,000 patients. Long after retirement, she continued to consult and treat occasional patients up till the time of her death.

Adalbert and Christa treating a patient with significant rib hump in the 70's at the institute in Sobernheim, Germany.

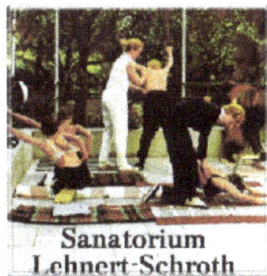

Sanatorium
Lehnert-Schroth

Schroth Into the '80s and '90s

While brace treatment developed and improved, the program lost its effectiveness after the Schroth Klinik was taken over by Asklepios in 1995. The groups of patients were too big for significant gains with only one therapist. In Barcelona, Dr. Manuel Rigo and Christa's son, Dr. Hans-Rudolf Weiss, (an MD and orthopedic specialist) improved the original program with the latest knowledge throughout the '90s.

59

Today Dr. Hans-Rudolf Weiss continues to carry on the research and treatment established by his mother and grandmother. The Schroth method is perhaps the most well-known scoliosis treatment. Schroth practitioners have different types of training, experiences and protocols. Sadly, Schroth is fractured. The most current version is Schroth Best Practice® (SBP) which comes directly from Dr. Weiss, the grandson of Katharina Schroth. Among its advantages are that it is less confusing to learn, focuses on improved muscle engagement with upright exercises as well as very important corrections in habits of everyday life to support the exercises. This is the method that I use in my practice.

For patients with very severe curves, the original Schroth exercises are still used. Barcelona Scoliosis Physical Therapy School (BSPTS) differs in that it does not include many of the newer, more user-friendly modifications. Teaching is also typically delivered differently (SBP is a short-term intensive treatment vs. BSPTS which has shorter sessions over a more extended period). Philosophies, teaching styles and support services vary from practitioner to practitioner.

Ask who and where a practitioner learned from. The extent of scoliosis treatment experience with Schroth is quite nuanced (full-

Lehnert-Schroth augmented classification:

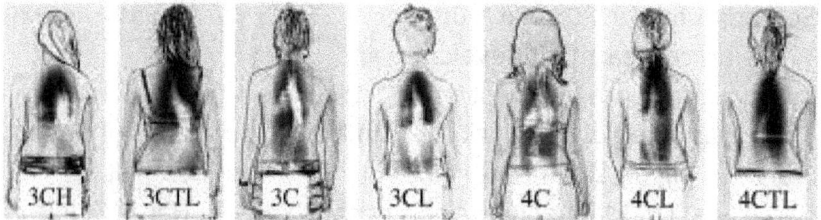

3CH   3CTL   3C   3CL   4C   4CL   4CTL

In the 70's Christa Lehnert-Schroth further developed the method and introduced a simple classification, which is still used today. Additionally, she discovered the importance of the lumbosacral counter-curve (4th Curve) for pattern specific postural correction

time or part-time practice). Also, ask about support services and follow-up. Information upfront will provide the best idea of what to expect. Hopefully, I have provided a lot of information to help you to choose the best treatment for yourself or your child.

7. SAGITTAL CURVES

As you recall from "What is Scoliosis" chapter 1, the sagittal curves are the front-to-back curves of the neck, upper back and lower back which normally should curve inward and outward to create a "spring-like" effect so as to allow the spine to absorb shock and impact. When these curves are out of alignment (too flat or too arched) the spine may be under increased stress. Any distortion of these front-to-back curves must be treated to reduce any stress to make the scoliosis curves easier to correct.

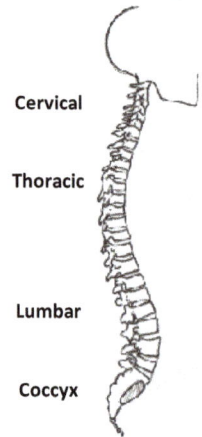

Cervical

Thoracic

Lumbar

Coccyx

Any good scoliosis program or brace should be designed to restore all of these curves to a more natural alignment. Tackling one dimension alone is not likely to get the best results.

In this X-ray you can see:

1. The cervical curve is too flattened.

2. The thoracic curve is too flattened.

3. The lumbar curve quickly loses its lordosis and leans back into a kyphosis at L2-3 and up.

4. The lower lumbar curve - is very curvy (Hyperlordotic).

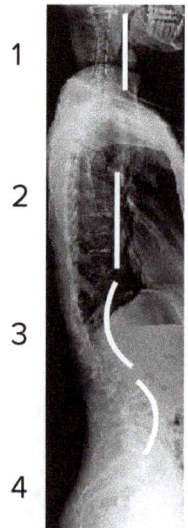

1

2

3

4

Text Neck / Forward Head Carriage / Scoli Neck

Text Neck: We spend too much time looking down at electronic devices which can lead to the loss of the normal neck curve and this loss of curve can create many neck issues and discomfort, as well as disc degeneration later in life. Many of us in the modern world and those of us who are diagnosed with scoliosis, typically have a flattened cervical curve that should be treated.

Notice in the second X-ray how flat/reversed the neck bones are stacked. This causes tension in the neck ligaments and muscles and creates a lack of shock absorption. Long-term effects include arthritis, pain and dysfunction.

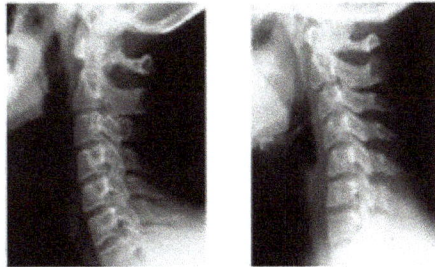

Normal Neck alignment / Flattened Neck Alignment

For some great "Text Neck" remedies and exercises, see Chapter 12 on "Exercise and Scoliosis".

Forward Head Carriage: Unlike those with "text neck," this posture is about the head being forward of the center of the body and creates stress on the neck and soft tissues. The skull weighs

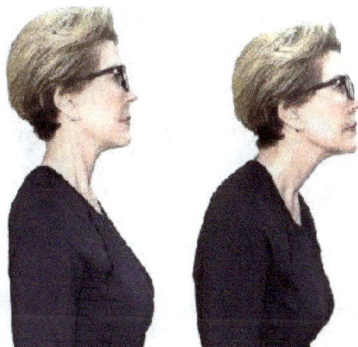

Normal neck alignment / Forward head carriage

about 10 pounds, so any forward movement of the head adds the weight of the skull exponentially into the neck (Skull 10 lbs. X inches forward = Lbs. of pressure on the neck).

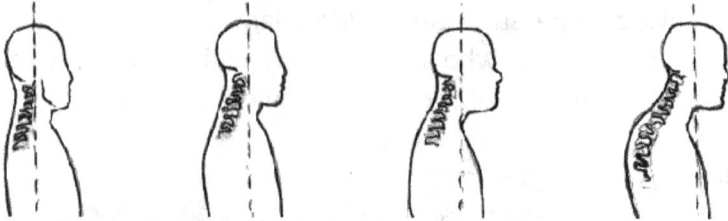
Normal neck alignment that slowly progresses to a forward head carriage

Cervical Scoliosis: An upper thoracic curve can creep up into the neck causing a head tilt or cervical scoliosis which is a relatively rare condition. Cervical scoliosis can also develop as a result of another medical condition, such as Klippel-Feil syndrome and Chiari Malformation. If someone is experiencing scoliosis-related neck pain or headaches it may be due to:

Stiff muscles, caused by a loss of motion in the spine.

A disruption to the flow of cerebrospinal fluid that passes through the spinal canal.

Combining chiropractic care, physical therapy, good ergonomics, home exercises and improving the neck's healthy curve, can greatly relieve pain. See Chapter 11 "What Should I Avoid?" for specific desk ergonomic setup information for work or school.

8. SURGERY

When a pediatrician or an adult's physician is concerned about scoliosis a referral will be made to a specialist such as an orthopedist or spine specialist. When visiting such a spine specialist, even in mild cases of scoliosis, the topic of surgery may come up. These conversations can be a bit scary for a child. If you are concerned about this, make sure your doctor knows your concerns before the visit if your child is present. It may be best not to have these conversations about surgery in front of your child until you as a family feel fully informed and have digested the information. After the consultation, have a conversation as a family before revisiting the doctor so that you and your child can ask any other follow-up questions.

Anybody performing scoliosis surgery today is assumed to be highly skilled and use the most effective techniques known. Getting a second or third opinion will help you gain more understanding and make a more informed decision. It is important to work with a surgeon who performs many surgeries each year. Please also read Chapter 14 "Choosing a Doctor".

There are many spinal surgery techniques and a variety of instrumentation alternatives including rods, screws, hooks, wires, etc., to reduce and stabilize the scoliosis curve. There are different types of fusions, fusion-less or growing rod types of procedures.

When should the surgery option be considered?

- When there is severe pain.
- The curve is causing extreme psychological distress.
- The curve is causing physical impairment.
- The curve is very large (greater than 40°) and the child is still growing and the curve is getting worse rapidly.
- The curve is continuing to progress greater than 45° even after growth has stopped.
- The curve is greater than 50º with severe trunk asymmetry.
- The curve is not idiopathic and has a clear cause that can be addressed with surgery.
- Bracing and therapy have failed to control the curve.

In some cases, more than one surgical procedure may be needed to achieve the best possible outcome. Your surgeon will consider all of the factors of your case and present you with the pros and cons of each viable procedure. This information will allow you to make an educated decision regarding which procedure you ultimately choose.

There are some fears that large scoliosis could impact the function of the heart and lungs. Studies show that there is only a small risk that those with scoliosis will ever develop these problems or have any issues with having children, working, or leading a productive life.

What are the Goals of Scoliosis Surgery?

- Prevent curve progression
- Straightening the spine as much as possible. More importantly, finding a balance of the torso and pelvis is the main goal, not to fully "straighten" a curve.
- All 3 dimensions of the spine should be addressed, meaning to straighten the curve itself, de-rotate the rotated vertebrae and restore the spine's front-to-back curves (sagittal) that are often disrupted in scoliosis.

How is Scoliosis Surgery Performed?

Fusing (joining together) or tethering the vertebrae along the curve with instrumentation (Rods, wires or other devices).

The particular surgical approach the surgeon selects is based on the following:

- Spinal maturity: is the patient's spine still growing?
- Degree of pain prior to surgery and the impact on the patient's health and lifestyle.
- Degree and extent of the curvature.
- The spine region(s) in which the curve occurs.
- Success or failure of previous treatment alternatives.
- Estimate of probable progression following surgery.

Posterior Approach	Anterior Approach	Thoracotomy
A straight incision is made along the midline of the back. This approach is used most often in the treatment of scoliosis and can be effective for all curve types This has been the standard in scoliosis surgery.	Usually used on the lower areas of the spine and involves shorter fusion levels. The lumbar spine can be approached through a frontal abdominal incision.	For surgery on the thoracic (middle) spine another approach may be by a lateral incision.

What are the types of surgery?

Regardless of the type of surgery you and your medical team decide to go with, some families involve a plastic surgeon to achieve the least visible scar possible whether it is a first-time surgery or a revision surgery. Discuss your options with your surgeon. Also, if there is a concern about any of the hardware having room under the skin, a skin expander may be used prior to surgery.

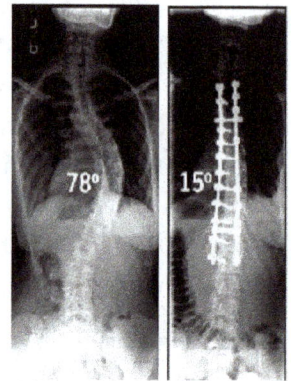

Figure 1: pre-op   Figure 2: Post-op

Fusion

This surgery permanently fuses two or more bones so that they form a solid area that no longer moves. Normally, this process takes months to completely heal. During the recovery period, the doctor will evaluate the fusion through imaging.

Posterior Fusion Types:

- Harrington Rod Procedure: First developed in the '60s and used as the most standard procedure until the early 90s. A steel rod extends from the bottom to the top of the curve. Hooks suspended from pegs are inserted into the bone to hold the rod. The vertebrae in between the hooks are then allowed to fuse. The Harrington rod is largely an older spinal fixation system. It allowed fixation at only two points. It required a body cast to be worn afterward for many months during the healing process. Modern rod fixation systems allow for multiple points of fixation making it much stronger. The newer systems also allow for better correction of deformity with little to no casting afterward.

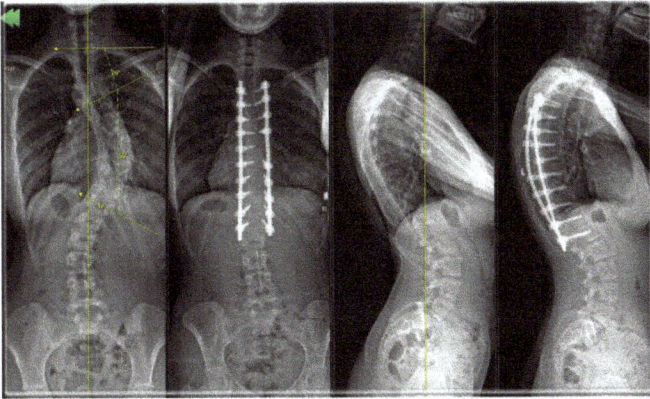

- Cotrel–Dubousset Instrumentation was Introduced in 1983 as a double-rod procedure. It uses a hybrid of techniques including more anchors, pedicle screws and wires in a cross-linked pattern which produces better curve correction and less instrument failure. Some patients not only got a better lateral and frontal curve correction but also correction of vertebral rotation and thus a good reduction in the cosmetic "rib bump". The post-surgical cast may still be needed.

- Luque L-rod or Luc Rod Instrumentation was introduced in the late 70s. It involves wiring and is a more difficult and potentially dangerous procedure due to the wire threaded through each vertebra near the spine. However, good results can be achieved. The main advantages are in maintaining the normal sagittal (front-to-back curvature) of the spine. It does not show good correction in the rotations of the spine, especially in the upper spine.

Anterior Fusion:
Anterior instrumentation surgery had been a choice of treatment for higher scoliosis curves because better correction can be obtained with shorter fusion levels (fewer bones involved). Initial enthusiasm for this surgery in expectation of decreased postoperative pain or patients' satisfaction with less surgical scar has faded out because the major blood vessel in the chest is at risk if a screw penetrates it and disruption of the chest cage during the surgery affects the lung function after surgery. Upper curves curve can be treated successfully with posterior instrumentation surgery without affecting lung function. In 2005, a study by Potter, Kuklo and Lenke in the "Spine Journal," compared anterior and posterior spinal fusion for upper curves and found that the posterior fusion technique demonstrated greater curve correction (62% vs. 52%) and greater rib hump correction (51% vs 26%). Recently, the anterior surgery has gone out of favor due to slightly less correction, longer surgery time and longer hospital stays compared to the posterior approach.

Fusionless, motion-sparing and growth-modulating spinal implants are the newest innovations in scoliosis surgery. Here are a few examples of the new technology:

Fusionless or "Growing Systems"
To avoid the complications of a fusion, the growing system method helps guide the spine as it grows, preventing the curve from worsening as the spine matures and eventually becomes ready for a fusion if needed. This surgery involves rods or staples that are anchored to the bones on only one side to guide the spine's curvature into a correction while a child grows. Once the child has finished growing, he or she may still require a more complete spinal fusion. These techniques are referred to as "anterior vertebral body growth modulation". These new options can avoid the complications of rigid fusion techniques and are

70

much less invasive. Good results have been shown in recent studies in growing children. The theory is that by putting constant pressure on a bone, it will grow more slowly and become more dense. By applying pressure on the outer side of a spinal curve to slow or stop the growth of the curve's outer side, the curve's inner side continues to grow normally. As the spine continues to grow, the curvature should reduce and the spine will become straighter.

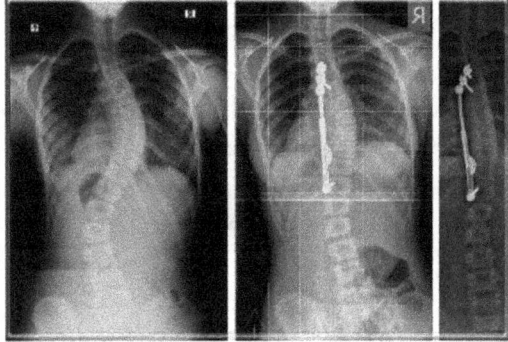

For now, these techniques are used with growing children but may be useful in idiopathic scoliosis in older populations in the future.

Types of Fusionless or (Growing System) Surgical Techniques:

- Vertebral tethering systems such as anterior scoliosis correction or anterior vertebral body tethering also called Vertebral Body Tethering (VBT): Implants are attached on one side of the spine to "hold" the bones as the other side is allowed to grow. Titanium screws are placed on the outside of the curve as a flexible rod cord is attached to each of the implants. When the cords are tightened, this corrects and straightens the spine from the outside of the curve. The curve(s) show an immediate improvement after surgery and continued improvement over time as the spine grows and "remodels".

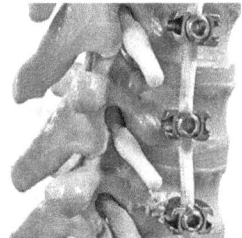

- Vertebral Body Stapling (VBS): Metal staples are implanted into the outside of a spinal curve on the front growth plates of the bones for growth modulation and curve stabilization and have proven to be effective.

Pros: Compared to spinal fusion, fusionless surgery has the potential benefit of retaining more spinal mobility.

Cons: This is a newer approach and long-term data about the risks and benefits are not yet available.

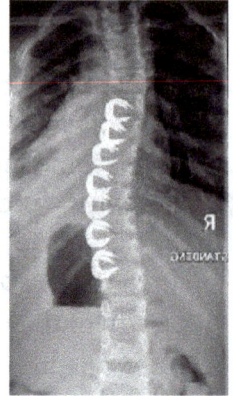

Growing Rods or Traditional Growing Rods (TGR)

For some children who are 2-10 years old, a "growing rod" may be utilized for correction without fusing the spine to allow growth of the spine and also allow the lungs to mature to full capacity. It usually involves rods attached to the top and the bottom of the spine only, with the rod running along the spine but not attached to each bone along its path. Growth-friendly techniques for the treatment of early onset scoliosis have greatly evolved since Harrington rods. Traditional growing rods require periodic surgical lengthening procedures under general anesthesia and are associated with a relatively high risk of complications.

Types of Growing Rods:

- Traditional growing rod: A metal rod attached to the spine is periodically lengthened by a simple procedure. It is usually attached to the spine on the top and then either attached to the spine or the hips on the bottom with the rod in between. This procedure involves the insertion of two rods. The difference between this and a full spinal fusion is that the screws are placed in the spine only at the top and the bottom. This allows continued growth of the spine. In the postoperative period, there is no casting or bracing necessary and the patient can return to full sports and other activities after about 6 months. The rods are generally lengthened every 6-9 months depending on the age of the child.

- Vertical Expandable Prosthetic Titanium Rib (VEPTR): The VEPTR device is different from the traditional growing rod in that it is attached to the ribs at the top of the device. It is then attached to the spine or the hips on the bottom. The innovation of the VEPTR provided treatment for the infant or child with thoracic insufficiency syndrome which is defined as the inability of the chest to support normal breathing or lung growth. If the chest cannot grow normally, the lungs cannot grow and life-threatening breathing problems may develop. The VEPTR has been designed to allow the rib cage to grow while controlling spinal deformity without fusion of the spine. Before this technique was developed, there was no effective treatment for the combination of chest wall deformity and scoliosis that created problems with lung growth and pulmonary function. With both devices, this lengthening procedure takes place under general anesthesia with a small incision to expose the device. Many children can go home the same day and can return to school after a couple of days and back to normal activities.

- A new posterior dynamic deformity correction device by ApiFx Ltd. from Israel is a less invasive surgery that allows some motion to remain in the spine and controls the curve over time. The device has a ratchet mechanism that allows the elongation of an expandable rod. The expandable rod is anchored to the spine with two screws on the inside (concavity) of the main curve. The ratchet mechanism gives immediate curve reduction and potential gradual postoperative curve correction by device elongation. This device was recently approved by the Federal Drug Administration (FDA) in the USA for the treatment of moderate scoliosis. The technique was associated with promising clinical and X-ray results. However, a high rate of serious adverse events within 2 years may be unacceptable for further clinical application, despite recent FDA approval.

- MAGnetic Expansion Control (MAGEC) "Magic Rods" (MAGnetic Expansion Control) System, a new surgical treatment approved by the FDA in 2014 for children with scoliosis who are still growing and was designed to reduce the number of repeated surgeries. This is a distraction-based growing rod technique that is non invasive when more lengthening is required during growth by using external magnets to control a rod implanted in the spine. The procedure is much like the traditional growing rod as it is attached to the ribs or the spine at the top and the spine or the pelvis at the bottom but the lengthening device is in the middle. With other growing rods, the patient must return for surgery to have the device lengthened every 6-9 months. With this system, the patient can have the lengthening done in the office without anesthesia by placing an external remote controller over the location of the magnet in a matter of minutes. An X-ray is done to confirm the amount of lengthening that was achieved. There is typically not any pain involved during the lengthening and there are no additional incisions or bandages. The child can get back to activities immediately. The visits to adjust the device are typically done every 3 months but this can vary based on the patient's age and curve. It decreases the chance of infection and the risks of anesthesia. Only a few facilities around the US currently offer this cutting-edge treatment. MAGEC rods are not appropriate for all children with severe spinal deformities and are not recommended for

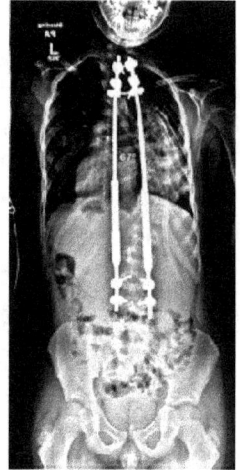

very young children or those who have finished growing. MAGEC rods may not be strong enough to lengthen a very stiff curve, so surgeons rarely do conversion operations (taking out growing rods or VEPTR devices and exchanging in MAGEC rods).

- Shilla Technique uses two rods that grow as the spine grows. Similar to a track and trolley system. The rods are placed but are partially fixed to the spine. This allows the system to "grow with the spine". Rod breakage can occur and this is a normal outcome. When this happens revision surgery is indicated. This is a newer technique being applied at leading centers across the country. Pedicle Screws are inserted at specific points in the spine. Screws in the center are holding the rods in place. Other screws allow for the spine to move and elongate at either end. The Shilla hardware hopes to minimize the number of surgeries needed during the growth period of a child, therefore minimizing the risk of infection and hardware failure.

Hybrid
Some surgeons will opt for a fusion of one area but a tethering or growing rod system for another area of the spine based on variations of the curves in the upper or lower parts of the spine.

Osteotomy
The affected bones are removed. A doctor will perform this procedure through either a front or back approach. Typically, doctors use this procedure to treat adults with rigid scoliotic curves, flat-back syndrome, children with large curves, or cases in which realignment is necessary following a previous spinal fusion.

Hemivertebrae Excision

Normally, spine bones are rectangular in shape. Hemivertebrae are wedge-shaped bones in the spine. This spinal deformity usually occurs before birth and often results in kyphosis or scoliosis as the patient grows. If the patient's condition is progressive and the patient exhibits a lack of balance, the hemivertebra bone should be removed. The surgeon will probably also implant rods and screws and more often than not, the patient will need to wear a brace for several months after the surgery.

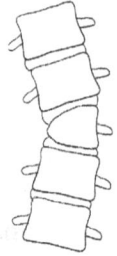

Video-Assisted Thoracoscopic Surgery (VATS)

Performed on patients with thoracic scoliosis curvature. The surgeon will need to temporarily deflate one of the lungs. Because of this, not all patients are candidates, as lung deflation is too risky for some. Certain curves will make access to the spine via VATS too difficult to be worth doing. During VATS, the doctor will make small incisions called portals in the side of the chest. The surgeon will utilize cameras, endoscopes and video monitoring devices to help make the procedure less invasive. After the procedure, the small incisions made during the surgery will be hidden by the patient's arm. The incisions are small and result in less scarring and a quicker recovery.

Thoracoplasty

Scoliosis patients usually have a prominent rib bump in the back (best seen bent over). This procedure's goal is to reduce the size of the rib bump. Usually, this involves the removal of as many as five ribs. Typically, this procedure is performed along with other scoliosis corrective surgeries, but it may be performed as a separate procedure. In some cases, the doctor will need to install a chest tube that will stay in for a day or two after the procedure is complete. This procedure is not very common today, as current advances have led to an improved rotational correction of the deformity. For an adolescent or young adult opting for scoliosis surgery today, by far the most commonly performed surgery is a spinal fusion.

Halo Gravity Traction

A method of gently stretching and straightening a severely compressed or curved spine. Children remain in the hospital the entire time they are in traction, typically three to eight weeks. After halo traction, children usually have fusion surgery. A surgeon attaches a lightweight metal ring (halo) to the child's skull with small pins. The halo is attached to a pulley system which is attached to the child's bed, wheelchair, or walker. Over the next several weeks, weight is added to the pulley to slowly straighten the curved or compressed spine. The pins will leave small lesions on the skin when they are first removed. The child will have small scars on his or her forehead but these generally fade and become less noticeable over time.

Possible Complications of All Procedures

- Infection. Antibiotics will be given to the patient to lessen this risk.

- Bleeding. Of course, some bleeding is expected. Some patients may require a transfusion for surgery. The patient or a family member may be asked to donate beforehand.

- If a bone graft was used, in some cases, patients will experience pain at the graft site after surgery.

- Nerve damage occurs in 1% of patients, with the risk highest in adults and most often causes muscle weakness. Paralysis is very rare. The surgeon will monitor nerve function during surgery to lessen the risk of neurological damage.

- Lung complications, like nerve damage, are rare. Healthy teenagers will rarely if ever have a lung issue after surgery. Fusion surgeries can restrict spinal growth of the fused areas which may negatively affect lung function and the potential for disk degeneration above and below a fusion.

- Loosening of instrumentation: This often occurs when the bones are not healing or fusing properly due to infection or other causes.

- Broken instrumentation: Instrumentation can break when the bones are not healing and the rods or screws fatigue. This process is somewhat like a paperclip you continuously bend until it breaks.

- Any fused vertebrae will lose some mobility, balance and strength which can cause back pain and chronic problems later on.

- Pseudoarthrosis: If the fusion fails to heal, a painful condition develops in which a false joint develops at the site.

- About 40% of patients with Harrington rods had "flat back" syndrome because the procedure typically eliminated normal front-to-back (sagittal) curves.

- In later years, the disks may collapse below the fusion and can cause pain.

- The rate of complications of spinal fusion surgery appears to increase with time after surgery.

- There is a risk of clinical failure (meaning the pain does not go away) despite a successful fusion.

- If a spinal fusion is done at a young age (younger than age 10 in girls or less than 12 in boys), it could leave less room for the lungs to develop or cause the child to have an unusually short trunk compared to the limbs. Revision (repeat) surgery may be needed in growing children and more surgeries equal more risk.

- One risk that can occur in a growing person is a "crankshaft deformity," which is a rotation of the spine. This is because the back of the spine is fused but the front of the spine keeps growing and causes rotation which can cause a new and different deformity.

Pros:

- Modern surgical approaches and instrumentation such as rods, screws, hooks and/or wires placed in the spine have made it easier to achieve better curvature correction and faster recovery times than in the past.

- Modern procedures tend to fuse fewer bones and maintain more movement than in the past.

- Surgery can be performed to correct all variations and types of scoliosis.

- Low risk of recurrence. Because of the way scoliosis surgery is typically performed, the spine isn't likely to become misaligned in the same area after surgery. However, it is still important to take precautions such as maintaining good posture.

- Because of advances in technology, surgery for scoliosis increasingly involves minimally invasive techniques done with smaller incisions, which usually means fewer risks and shorter recovery times.

- Less-invasive surgical techniques also reduce the risk of damage to nearby parts of the spine, including adjacent discs and nerves. In some instances, smaller hardware may be used to further ease the stress on other parts of the spine.

- Most patients respond well to surgery for scoliosis, often experiencing fewer instances of spine-related pain.

Do the Instruments or Rods Break?

They can, but it is uncommon. Most rods are made of titanium, cobalt-chromium, or stainless steel depending on your surgeon and your case. If a rod breaks, it is a sign that a portion of the bone and instrument did not fuse properly. If there is no solid fusion, the rod will be repeatedly stressed over time. No matter how strong your rod is, repetitive stress like this will lead to eventual breaks.

Removal of Rods

A surgeon may decide to remove spinal instrumentation if:

- The pain is relentless
- The hardware has loosened
- The hardware has become infected
- The hardware is irritating other tissues such as muscles, organs, nerves, or the spinal cord.

If the spinal instrumentation is causing pain after surgery, your surgeon may recommend not removing it. Why? Because undergoing a second surgery puts the patient at risk for additional complications and removing the instrumentation alone may not eliminate the pain.

Understanding the clear risks and benefits of undergoing a second surgery will help you make the best decision. The decision is far more important than the incision.

A surgeon may refer to this second surgery as a revision surgery or a reconstruction surgery. These terms are frequently interchangeable, but there are slight differences between them.

- Revision surgery means removing or exchanging spinal instrumentation.
- Reconstruction surgery means rebuilding the spine.

Spinal surgery to remove instrumentation is not typically considered an emergency unless there is a risk of injury to the spinal cord or nerves by not doing the surgery. This may occur if the instrumentation has moved and is putting pressure on the nerves.

How Much Will Surgery Cost?
The exact cost of a specific surgery is hard to determine. Costs depend on a variety of factors, such as:

- How many days you are in the hospital.
- Types of material used for the surgery.
- The bone graft material used for the surgery, if any.
- The surgeon's fees
- The anesthesia fees
- Medications
- Aftercare/physical therapy/home care
- Any complications that lead to an extended hospital stay.

Make sure that you discuss your plans with your provider first as surgery can become costly. Please read Chapter 17 "Resources" to find financial aid information.

Not every patient will qualify for surgery. If the patient smokes cigarettes, has a spinal infection or tumor, or suffers from allergies to the surgical materials used during the procedure, then other treatments may work better rather than surgery.

Getting Ready for Surgery
Spinal fusion with spinal instrumentation is major surgery. The patient will undergo many tests to determine the nature and exact location of the curve. These tests are likely to include X-rays, magnetic resonance imaging (MRI), computed tomography scans (CT scans), or other scans of your urinary system. The patient will have blood and urine tests and possibly an electrocardiogram. In some rod instrumentation, the patient may be placed in traction or an upper body cast to stretch contracted muscles before surgery. Skin spacers may be used to prepare the skin for the surgery. Blood may be needed for the patient during surgery so a donation by the patient or by a family member may be needed. A brace may be worn before surgery to stabilize the spine and a brace after surgery may be required to secure the fused areas after surgery. These are things to discuss with your surgeon. Another topic to discuss would be the weight of the patient. Since some lose weight after surgery it may be recommended to put on some weight before the surgery.

What is the Recovery Timeline After Surgery?
After surgery, the patient will be on bed rest. A catheter may be inserted so that the patient can urinate without getting up. Vital signs are monitored and the patient's position is changed frequently so that bedsores do not develop. Recovery from spinal instrumentation can be a long process. Movement is severely limited for a period of time. In certain types of instrumentation, the patient is put in a cast to allow the instruments and bones to be held protected until healing takes place for as long as six to eight months. Some patients will need to wear a brace after the cast is removed. During recovery, the patient is taught breathing exercises, self-care and strengthening and range of motion

exercises. The length of the hospital stay depends on the age and health of the patient, as well as the specific problem that was corrected. The patient can expect to remain under a physician's care for many months. The first 4 weeks after surgery is when you need to be mindful of infection. Bathing may be restricted for the first 2 weeks.

Post-surgery, some symptoms to be aware of include:
- Fever (101 degrees or higher)
- Expanding redness at the incision
- Increasing back pain
- Change in the amount, appearance, or odor of drainage.

If these signs appear, contact the surgeon immediately. Any stitches or staples will usually be removed about 2 weeks after surgery. If the wound has completely healed, bathing or swimming may be allowed.

Medication Transition
If an opioid pain medication is used, the prescription will typically include instructions for how to gradually wean off the medication over a few weeks. If no medicine or specific instructions are given, ask the surgeon and/or pharmacist for recommendations. Proper medication management is important. Over or under-medicating both have risks. Be alert for allergies if a drug has never been taken before and remember, pain is counterproductive to healing so follow your instructions carefully.

X-ray and MRI after Surgery
Most metal implants used in spine fusions are made of either stainless steel or titanium. Titanium is a non-magnetic material that is not affected by the magnetic field of MRI. The risk of implant-based complications is very low and MRI can be safely used in patients with implants. Also, patients wonder if the

instrumentation could set off airport metal detectors and require them to undergo additional screening. The most basic answer for individuals undergoing spinal surgery is: no, this scenario is unlikely. "Magic Rods" have magnets and are therefore not able to be in an MRI machine.

Exercise after Surgery
Patients usually begin to feel a little stronger each day but need to be aware of infection risks and medication safety issues. A return to full activity, sports, or exercise may take as long as 6 months to a year to be sure the areas have healed.

Post-surgical clients must wait 8-12 weeks before exercise and must have the doctor's permission. The work will be mostly isometric and the goals are now very different. Regular low-impact exercises will help to stretch and strengthen the muscles around the spine. Gentle and regular exercise will help the patient feel better physically and mentally. Always follow the guidelines of the healthcare provider.

Recommended post-surgery activities include:
* Swimming
* Gentle stretching / Pilates
* Stationary bicycle
* Elliptical
* Walking

Any intense exercise such as heavy lifting, bending and twisting are all off-limits, at the beginning. A regular full sports and exercise program may have to wait for 6 months or longer for recovery and rehabilitation to be completed.

What exercises should you avoid after scoliosis surgery?
Exercises that involve traction, high impact, extension, flexion, rotation, or side bending of the fused areas of the spine or neck, can place pressure on the hardware, the spinal discs and the now hyper-mobile joints above and below the spinal fusion site. These should be avoided as much as possible. Instead, focus on stability in the areas above and below the fusion and more frequent low-impact exercises after scoliosis surgery.

Post Fusion Surgery Exercise Guide
This book provides content related to physical and, or mental health issues. As such, the use of this book implies your acceptance of this disclaimer.

Always seek the advice of a qualified health care provider with any questions regarding a medical condition or treatment and obtain clearance before undertaking a new health care regimen and never disregard professional medical advice or delay in seeking it because of something you have read in this book, or elsewhere. No material in this book is intended to be a substitute for professional medical advice, diagnosis, or treatment. The material, including but not limited to, text, graphics, images and other material contained in this book is for informational purposes only. If pain, swelling, loss of function, numbness, tingling, or decreased range of motion are present or develop, consult your doctor.

Week 1: Start Rehabilitation and Exercise
You will focus on:
- Rest
- Pain management and weaning from pain medicines.
- A healthy diet and plenty of fluids.
- Getting back to independent self-care.

Follow the doctor's guidance at all times. You may be advised to start short walks very soon in the days after surgery and continue short but frequent walks, increasing the amount and length of the walks as tolerated. Always be aware of surroundings to avoid falling risk and be aware of posture and normal spinal movement front to back and not side-to-side. It is normal to be nervous and afraid to exercise after surgery. Talk to your doctor and perhaps ask for a referral to talk to others who have had your surgery. Talk to your physical therapist and always insist that you feel comfortable and trust your therapist to increase your confidence and healing.

Transitioning during daily life and exercises will be challenging and you need to learn how to "log roll" the body to the side and use a one-arm push-up to get up. Do not roll up or down.

Stretching before each walk is advised. For all stretches, go gently and never to the point of pain. It is important to stretch the hamstrings and quadriceps as well as the spine to prevent adhesions or scar tissue around nerves and muscles.

Quadriceps Stretches
Performing a stretch while side lying will prevent any spinal bending or balance issues at first. Capture your ankle and gently pull while tucking your pelvis under and lengthening the knee away from the front of your hip. Breathe and hold for 10-30 seconds on each side. Remember, log roll to switch sides.

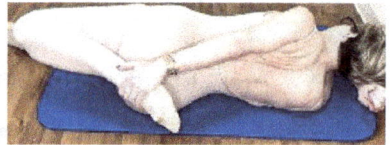

Hamstring Stretches

(Can irritate Sciatica. If electrical pain goes up the leg or spine, this is an urgent medical situation - stop and call your doctor).

Lie on your back and support your neck with a towel or pillow if needed. Find the neutral spine position (described later) and maintain it while slowly straightening one leg and pressing the heel toward the ceiling using a band, towel, or a Pilates ring, etc.

Modification: supporting the back of the thigh with both hands. Hold for 10 to 30 seconds, relax and repeat 3 times. Repeat with the other leg.

The goal is to maintain a neutral spine. Do not flatten the low back if possible during the stretch.

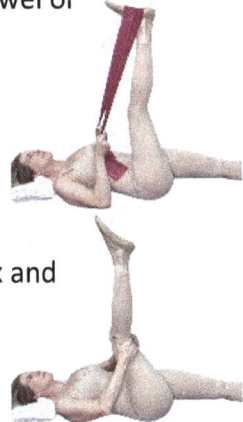

Nerve Stretches

Nerve stretches (mobilization) should be done in a "flossing" way without bouncing or long holding. The purpose is to reduce scar tissue from occurring around the nerves. Gently perform the previous hamstring stretch and release. Perform these "pumps" a few times only to your comfort level. To be done daily or as prescribed by your doctor.

Gastrocnemius/Soleus Stretch

Stand facing the wall, hands on the wall, step one leg back bend the knee to stretch the soleus or straighten the knee to stretch the gastrocnemius. Lean into the wall keeping the heel on the floor for 30 seconds.
Do this for each leg.

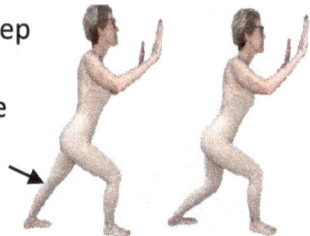

Piriformis Stretches

These stretches involve rotation of the knee, stop if pain is felt.

1. Figure four stretch: Supine, cross 1 ankle over the opposite knee and draw knee to chest
2. Pull the knee towards the chest and then towards the opposite shoulder
3. Pigeon stretch on the floor
4. Pretzel stretch cross one ankle outside the opposite knee and use the elbow to lift and twist away from the bent knee
5. Foam Roll: seated long ways on the roller, cross one ankle over the opposite knee, lean to the bent knee side of the glute and roll back and forth avoiding bone, only massaging the muscle.

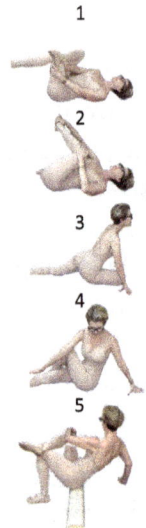

Psoas Stretch

Place the foam roller under the lowest part of the pelvis in a horizontal position (NOT in the low back!) hold behind one knee and pull to the chest as the opposite leg extends away and opens the front of the hip.

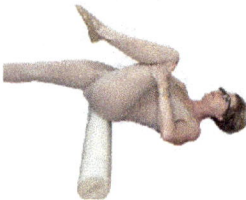

Pectorals / Chest Stretches

- Doorway or corner stretches with hands at 3 variable levels: eye level, shoulder level, chest level

- Overhead towel/band stretch make sure not to arch the back

- Foam roller supine arm circles or "hold up" position: lying lengthwise on a 6X36" foam roller.

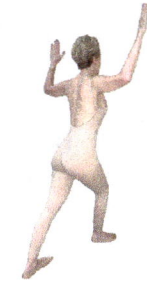

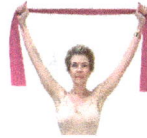

Weeks 1-9: Stabilization Exercises

After a few weeks, you are now focusing on:

- Increasing activity and endurance.

- Returning to school three to six weeks after surgery.

- Returning to normal life except for activity/sports restrictions.

- Being off all pain medicine.

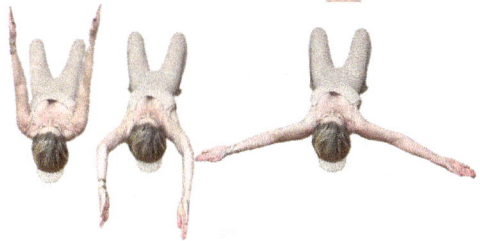

The purpose is to activate the muscles around the spine and pelvis that become weak and lead to an unstable structure. Working the small and deep stabilizer muscles will reap huge rewards even if they seem simple or too easy. It is vital to start slowly and build from there. The following exercises focus on moving the limbs but holding still in the torso, with no rocking, bending, or arching of the spine.

First, we must learn to hold the spine in a "neutral position". A neutral spine/pelvis is imperative to maintain the integrity of the curves of the spine and to allow the muscles to provide stability.

We will learn this in all positions and use it in each exercise regardless of recovery status.

How to find a neutral spine while lying on your back
Two ways to find neutral. Support your neck and or low back with a towel or pillow if needed.
1. Pelvic Positioning: Hook lying position (lie on your back with knees bent and feet flat on the floor, arms at sides). The two front hip bones and pubic bone should be horizontally level (neutral pelvis). This alignment forms a triangular shape and a small amount of space between your spine and the floor.
2. Thoracic/Lumbar Positioning: Hook lying position. The ribs and tailbone should be down on the mat with all the vertebrae between the ribs and tailbone relaxed into a soft natural "arch". Imagine enough space in the small of your back for ladybugs to crawl through (see photo). If you are lying down in this position correctly, your pelvis should feel level and your ribs should feel slightly contracted together as if you are tightening a corset to keep the ribs down.

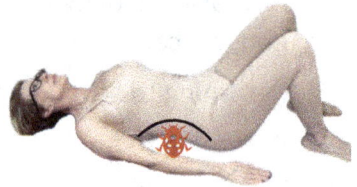

How to find a neutral spine in a side-lying position
Stack the hips and reach the top leg lengthwise (pulling the hip away from the armpit) to create a small space under the waistline of the downside called a "mouse house".

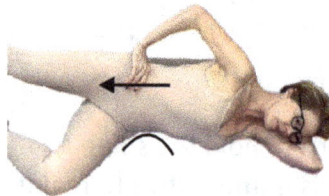

How to find a neutral spine in face down (prone) position

The pubic bones and front hip bones align in the front with the 10th rib. Reach out thru the crown of the head to avoid hyperextension, reach out of the spine and engage abs up into the spine, a small roll or pillow under the belly or pelvis if needed to support the low back.

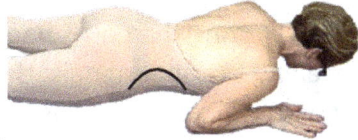

How to find a neutral spine in a plank position

Legs hip distance apart, tuck the tailbone slightly and abs pulled up into the spine. Imagine a slight rainbow shape of the low back. This position is an "overcorrection" to support the low back from overly arching and becoming prone to injury. Press away so that the shoulder blades aren't "winging".

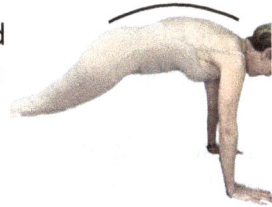

How to find a neutral spine while seated

The pelvic alignment can be visualized as a "pelvic bowl" that must remain upright. This can be best felt by sitting on a hard surface and rocking the pelvis back and forth. When the pelvic bones "sits" bones are felt to be their most prominent or "boney" the pelvic bowl should be in its upright position.

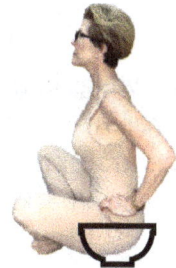

How to find a neutral spine while standing or kneeling

Align the upper core with the lower core as if the torso and pelvis were columns and need to be stacked, shoulders down, head over shoulders. Imagine that upright bowl as discussed in the seated position.

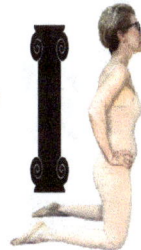

Pelvic Tilt/Tuck

Hook lying position (lie on your back with knees bent and feet flat on the floor, arms at sides). Support your neck with a towel or pillow if needed. Press the low back into the floor by tilting the pelvis backward and engaging the abdominals. Hold 10 seconds, release, 3-5 reps. (knees to the chest can accomplish the same stretch, make sure to always capture the knees behind the knees rather than on top of the shins to protect the knees).

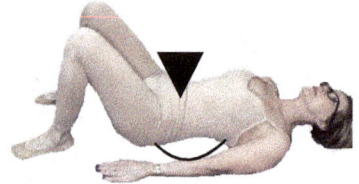

Pelvic Bridge

Hook lying, neutral spine. Put a small ball or rolled-up towel between the knees, inhale to prepare, exhale while engaging the abdominals and lift the hips only to the point that the 12th rib is still down. Remain neutral (don't crush the imaginary ladybugs in the small of your back). Inhale and hold as you imagine length in the spine, exhale and lower down over the neutral space/ladybugs as your tailbone touches the mat before the low back. 5-10 reps.

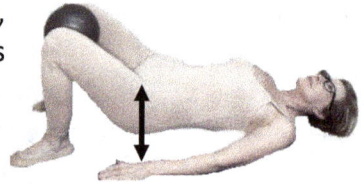

Pelvic Bridge Variations

Use a pelvic bridge as previously outlined for all of the following exercises. Relax shoulders, contract abdominals, keep the ribs down and breathe.

Progress to more challenging stability: Ffeet on a foam roller, a Bosu Ball®, a ball or a wobble board, etc.)

- Traction/Arm Float: hinge the hips up and hold as you float the arms over the head behind you. Lower hips, <u>then</u> return arms down to sides. Do this slowly, deliberately and with the sense of length and traction effect on the spine. This should feel like a stretch along the entire spine and armpits. 5-10 reps.

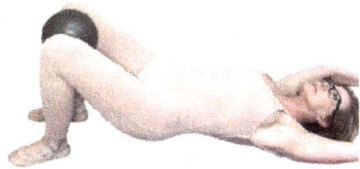

- Stability/Single Leg: hinge the hips up and without letting the hips lose a level position, slowly lift one foot off of the floor 1-2 inches only and stabilize the pelvis and low back. Lower the foot back to the floor and repeat on the other side without lowering the hips. Don't allow hips to become unlevel. 5-10 reps.

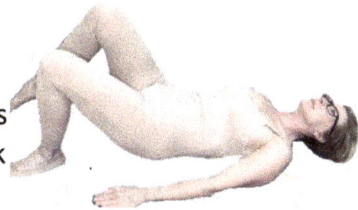

- Exercise Ball Bridges: an advanced stabilization exercise that introduces unpredictable movement that must be responded to (the movement of the ball). Lie on your back with both feet resting on top of a small exercise ball with knees bent and arms relaxed to the sides. The feet are on the ball about hip distance apart or together. Find the neutral spine position and hold it while slowly tightening the buttock muscles to lift the buttocks off the floor

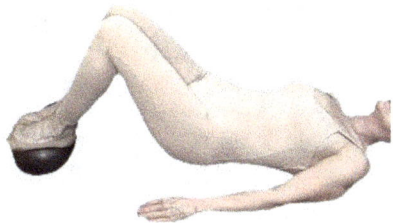

93

anywhere from 2-6 inches. Monitor the ball at all times to avoid loss of control. 5-10 reps.

Spinal Extension/McKenzie Type Exercises
Caution with your range of motion. Work within neutral and venture carefully into flexion or extension and monitor the reaction. Careful with spinal conditions such as spondylolisthesis, fused areas, facet syndrome and osteoporosis.

Swimming
Lie on your stomach with arm is placed on the floor elongated in front of you, leg slightly apart, long neck, gauge abdominals and roll back the shoulder blades. Lift 1 arm, rest and then opposite arm. Lift 1 long leg up, rest, then the opposite side.

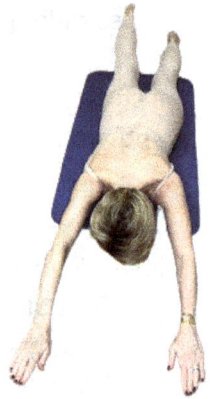

- Graduate to 1 arm and opposite leg lifting simultaneously then switch.
- Graduate to all limbs lifting at once and "swim" quickly for 30-60 sec.
- Graduate to lifting the head along with limbs and "swim" for 30-60 sec.

Always monitor any low back pain and don't focus on how high the limbs are being lifted but on the length of the limbs. Keep the face looking downward and the abdominals engaged. Focus on where the extension is happening in the back: upper or lower back or more plank-like with no bending of the spine.

Modifications:

- Rest your forehead on a towel or pillow.
- Arms bent into a "W" shape of elbows
- Just lift both bent elbows up and down - NO legs
- Small roll or pillow under the belly or pelvis if needed to support the low back.

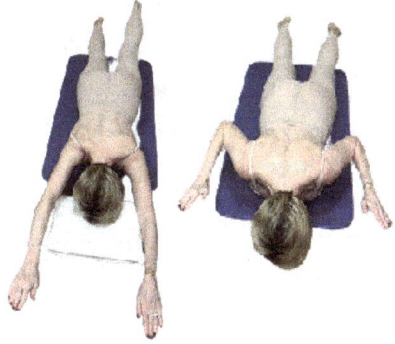

Cobra

Lie on your stomach with hands and bent elbows placed on the floor along the torso, legs slightly apart and long neck, engage your abs and roll back the shoulder blades. Inhale to press into arms and hands to lift the chest to approx. lower rib level, exhale to release. 2-3 reps.

Always monitor any low back pain and don't focus on how high the torso is being lifted, but how elongated the body can remain. Focus on where the extension is happening in the back. It may be focused on the upper or lower back or try to work more plank-like with no bending of the spine. Keep the face looking downward and the abdominals engaged.

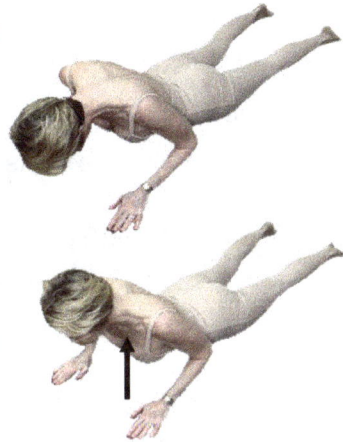

Cross Crawl

Kneeling on all 4's position. Visualize the torso as a table and strive to maintain complete stability. Hands directly under shoulders and knees directly under hips. Correct all the sagittal curves and roll the shoulders back, engage the core. Lift 1 arm directly out in front of you and return, then lift the opposite arm and return. Then lift 1 leg directly behind you while maintaining level hips and return, then lift the opposite leg and return. Progress to combine opposite arm and leg, keeping hips level, staying within the frame, abdominals engaged and spine long. Do NOT allow the abs to disengage or allow the spine to arch or rotate.

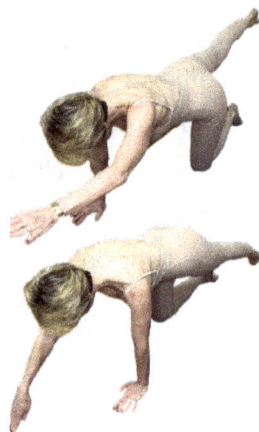

- Sustained lift with touch-down / lift
- Advanced: Lift the same arm as the leg on the same side, reverse.

5-10 reps. Modification: Perform over a properly sized ball to support your torso. An ottoman, toy box, or other small boxes may work.

Core Exercises

Perform basic ab/core exercises modified for back pain: Legs reach higher, keep neutral if possible with no pain, or imprint the spine to the mat. In the table top position, bring your knees closer to your chest or cross the ankles if back pain occurs. Find ways to work the core without flexion of the spine.

Abdominal Cross Crawl

Hook lying to lift one leg at a time up into a "tabletop" position, maintain a neutral spine, contract abs and inhale to lower one bent leg at a time towards the floor then lift with an exhale. Alternate legs and add the opposite arm lifting upwards as well. Maintain core and breathing. 5-10 reps.

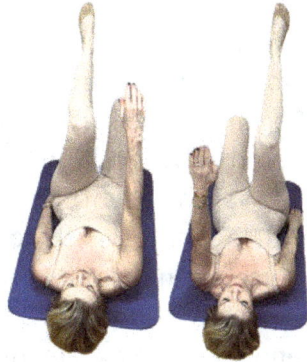

Table Top Knee Drifts

Hook lying to lift one leg at a time up into a "tabletop" position, maintain neutral (if pain; imprint the spine to the mat, pillow up the tailbone or draw knees closer to chest and cross ankles) keep the abdominals engaged and hips "nailed to floor" inhale allowing both bent legs to drift to one side, exhale returning legs to center and reverse. Modify distance with pain or pelvic instability. 5-10 reps.

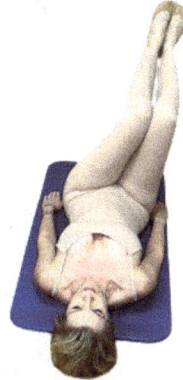

Legs Lower Lift

Lying face up, hook lying to lift one leg at a time up into straight legs up position, maintain neutral (Beginner: small pillow or hands under hips for tucked pelvis position to give low back support, knees slightly bent). Relax shoulders, inhale as legs drift slightly away and back up with an exhale. Do not allow the lower back to overarch, make movements as small as needed to control the lower back position. 5-10 reps.

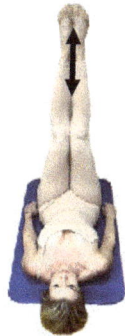

Legs side-to-side

Lying face up, hook lying to lift one leg at a time up into straight legs up position, maintain neutral (Beginner: small pillow or hands under hips for tucked pelvis position to give low back support, knees slightly bent). Relax shoulders, inhale as both legs drift slightly to the side (one leg becomes shorter than the other) then back to center with an exhale, drift to the opposite side and back to center with an exhale. Alternate side - center - side. Hips will not lift and the spine will not rotate. 5-10 reps.

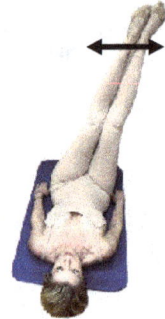

Corkscrew *(Combination of the previous 2 exercises)*

Lying face up, hook lying to lift one leg at a time up into straight legs up position, maintain neutral (Beginner: small pillow or hands under hips for tucked pelvis position to give low back support, knees slightly bent). Relax shoulders, inhale as both legs drift slightly to the side then slightly down and away around to the other side and back up to the center with an exhale. (as if starting at the top of a clock and making a full clock circle). Reverse direction each time and do not let hips lift, keep the hips pressed into the mat, when stopping before reversing direction, stop firmly and make the abdominals contract with a strong exhale. Avoid momentum. 5-10 reps.

Balance Activities

Always use a stable point to hold onto for any balance activity. Make sure surfaces are slip-proof and that you monitor getting on or off of any unstable prop. Do NOT attempt to close your eyes during balance activities; this may cause dizziness and be too challenging. Focus on the length of the spine and the natural curves of the spine and breathe into concave areas. Contract the abdominals and always keep safety at the forefront of your mind.

Full or Half Foam Roller

Stand and balance with slightly bent knees. Option to stand on a single leg for more challenge.

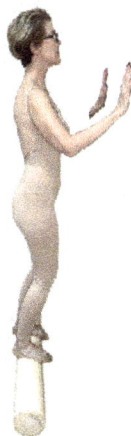

Bosu® Ball

Stand and balance on the dome with feet hip distance apart and slightly bent knees, single leg option on the dead center of Bosu. *It is NOT recommended to flip the Bosu flat side up. A warning is printed on the Bosu ball. If you attempt, be SURE to have stable assistance while getting on and off as it will tilt. Use non-slip material.*

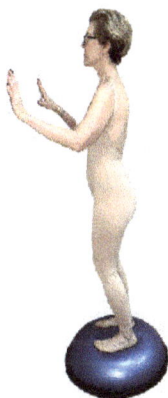

Wobble Board

Stand and balance with feet hip distance and slightly bent knees. Option to stand on a single leg for more challenge on the dead center of the board. Be cautious while getting on and off, as it will tilt. Use non-slip material.

Pilates 1st position / Turned out
Rise up onto your toes and balance (Arms out or up).

Graduating from Rehab Exercises
Six weeks to one year after surgery, activity restrictions may remain if activity puts too much stress on the healing bones and may prevent them from fusing properly.

These restrictions will ease as the year progresses and you are able to engage in high-impact sports, physical education, heavy lifting and aggressive twisting, or stretching of the spine.

One year+ after surgery:

- There are no restrictions on activities or sports.
- You will return for check-ups based on the surgeon's suggestion.
- The risk of developing complications is now very low.

Typically the patient will need to wait about one year after surgery to be sure the fusion is stable. A new set of X-rays to check the hardware placement and stability and a letter of clearance from an orthopedic surgeon are required before embarking on an exercise program.

Total fusion to the lowest lumbar bones (L5, sacrum, or pelvis) will have more restrictions.

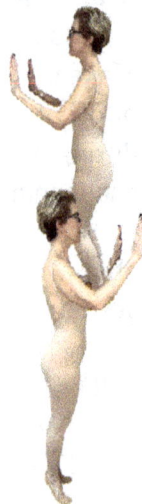

- Wedging or pillowing as performed in the Schroth technique in general is ok as needed on the convex side only. Go gently and monitor the reaction.
- In general, the only limitation is decreased mobility.
- No hanging or traction exercises since you don't want to damage the hardware.
- Less shifting exercises.
- Focus on corrective breathing into the concavities, symmetry and length to create a "cylinder" of a strong torso.
- If possible use a ball instead of a chair for better core training when seated.
- Safety at all times and reduce any risk of falling at home, work and the gym, etc.

Pain

You should not feel pain during exercise at all. If there is any pain, stop immediately. Gentle muscle pain after two days is normal in the areas that you worked. If soreness limits walking or other daily activities due to pain, either the exercise was performed incorrectly, too intensely or that exercise is not for you. Always be aware of your posture and body alignment by checking yourself in the mirror and/or relying on a good instructor.

- Start with one gentle exercise
- Start with low repetitions
- Wait for two to three days
- If you feel no pain at all after two to three days, continue with the first exercise and add a second
- Wait for another two to three days
- If you feel no pain at all, add a third exercise to your routine

- Wait for another two to three days
- If you feel no pain at all, add a fourth exercise and so on ... If you do feel pain, which at its maximum should be no more than gentle muscle pain, you will now be aware that a particular exercise is to be avoided.

Years after surgery:

- There are no restrictions on activities or sports.
- You will return for check-ups based on the surgeon's suggestion for quite a while - you should keep these appointments to monitor your hardware and fusions.
- Female patients can expect normal pregnancies but should monitor ligament "relaxing" during pregnancy and nursing due to Relaxin hormone.
- Scoliosis may be genetic so check your children.
- Keep a healthy lifestyle with exercise, maintain a good weight, remain active and avoid all tobacco.

9. BRACING

The goals of any brace should be:

- Straighten the spine as much as possible
- Balance the curves as much as possible
- Balance the torso and pelvic areas
- Improve any pulmonary disorders
- Improve back pain
- Improve the quality of life
- Improve psychological and cosmetic issues

What If My Doctor Tells Me To Watch And Wait?
This was discussed in Chapter 2 "Diagnosis Scoliosis" but I want to discuss this again. This topic comes up frequently. Parents visit an orthopedist or pediatrician when they first discover that their child has scoliosis. Most of these consultations involve discussions of surgery and how a brace won't help. Doctors frequently suggest a "watch and wait" plan with follow-up imaging in a few months. Watching and waiting should include constant monitoring of the situation and acting quickly if the curve appears to be worsening. If a child is still growing, it is possible that the curve could progress substantially. This can happen very quickly. There _are_ cases of children having small curvatures remaining stable or even spontaneously correcting, but it is generally a huge risk to watch and wait and do nothing, while so much growth is happening so quickly. Valuable time is wasted with the "watch and wait" plan, especially if the child's curve is between 20º-40º and the child is still growing.

A proactive approach can include:

- A second opinion
- Frequent monitoring of the scoliosis
- Scoliosis-specific postural exercises (SSPE)
- Bracing - do your research

Can All Types of Scoliosis Benefit From a Brace?
Although this book focuses primarily on idiopathic scoliosis (unknown cause) and specifically on children, I will also discuss bracing for adults. Most often, bracing is done for idiopathic scoliosis but other types of scoliosis are non-idiopathic, such as neuromuscular or congenital. These non-idiopathic types don't typically respond well to bracing. There is little data on bracing for these cases, but the surgical complications are high, so when non-surgical treatment is an option it should be seriously considered since there are encouraging (although infrequent) cases of success with bracing in non-idiopathic scoliosis.

Other Uses for a Brace
Braces can be used on a growing child to correct scoliosis, to protect the back during healing after scoliosis surgery, or with adults to prevent curve progression and provide support, or help with pain. Specialized braces can also be made for people who have an instability of the spine, a kyphosis (round back), or a "flat back."

How Do I Know If I Need a Brace?
Today, braces are strongly recommended for idiopathic curvatures between 20º-40º in children who are still growing. A growing child will need regular brace monitoring and may outgrow the brace at some point and need a new one. When the bones stop growing the use of braces is usually discontinued. This is discussed later since there is some controversy. Some adults

104

may wear a brace to halt curve progression, relieve pain, or remedy some other type of spinal issue. I will discuss adult bracing later on as well. Just because you are fully grown it does not mean you cannot still use a brace!

Types of Braces

Brace treatment protocols, types and quality vary. Treatment must be individualized for each person, using the highest level of care, skill, quality, technique and follow-up. Incorrect design can have a long-lasting negative impact on the person's quality of life. It is important to do your research and find the best brace for your situation.

There are several types of braces on the market (see below). These braces all have different biomechanical corrective principles, with varying effectiveness in correcting or halting the progression of curvatures. Remember that 3 planes of the spine need correcting. The frontal plane = side-to-side curves, the

sagittal plane = front-to-back curves and the transverse plane =
the rotations.

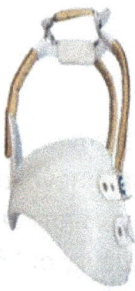
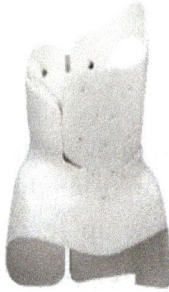
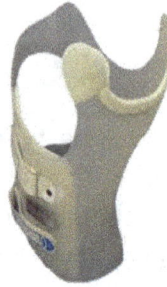
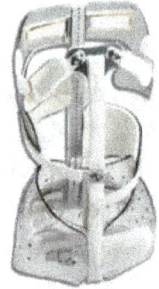

Milwaukee   Boston   Chêneau   Lyon

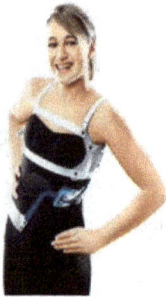
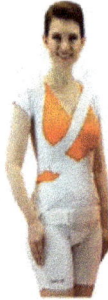
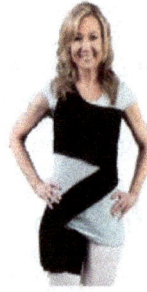
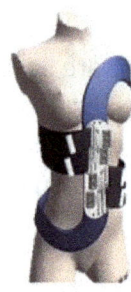

TriaC   SpineCor   ScoliSMART   Flexpine

The curves must be pushed into a correction but allowing room to
breathe and allowing the muscles to work and not atrophy or
weaken due to compression. The brace should be lightweight and
manageable to wear.

To give you an unbiased window into the world of scoliosis
bracing you need to know about the Scoliosis Research Society
(SRS) and the International Society for Scoliosis Orthopedic and
Rehabilitation Treatment (SOSORT). The SOSORT organization
mandated a brace classification study to provide definitions of all
brace types and a visual catalog. The study is well-rounded and
contains contributions from many sources. It would be helpful for
you to do your own research.

106

Let's outline the general types of braces and some specific braces as well.

- Asymmetrical: A brace that pushes on the curves and rotations but allows space (called "blowouts") in other areas.

- Symmetrical: In very general terms, a symmetrical brace may simply squeeze a scoliotic curve around the torso, like a corset. Padding may be used to create pressure in specific areas. These braces generally tend to cause more discomfort than asymmetrical braces.

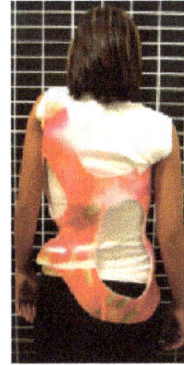
Asymmetrical Brace

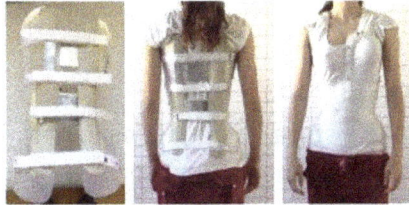
Symmetrical Brace

- Rigid: Usually made of plastic and ranges from flexible, to semi-rigid, rigid, to highly rigid. The rigid brace causes significantly more problems with heat, as well as difficulties with putting it on and taking it off, as compared to an elastic or flexible brace.

- Casting Bracing: This is done for infants and toddlers with congenital scoliosis or idiopathic scoliosis. The child has a wet plaster cast applied to the trunk on a table that allows control and correction of the curves. Casting is changed about every 8 weeks. Each new cast gradually increases the correction. The cast is made of fiberglass and is usually applied under general anesthesia. Correction is usually achieved by around 18 months of age. Casting is followed up with removable brace treatment to maintain the correction. Except for bathing and exercise, the new removable brace is to be worn all the time, usually for 2 to 3 years. The child is then weaned off the brace, provided that the correction of the curvature has been made and the spine is stabilized.

- Soft/Elastic: Popular in the early 2000s but now rarely used. Primarily composed of elastic straps. Examples are the ScoliSMART™ Activity Suit and the Spinecor® brace. People often have difficulties with putting it on and going to the bathroom. A current study shows that the failure rate of soft braces is significantly higher than that of rigid braces. Other soft

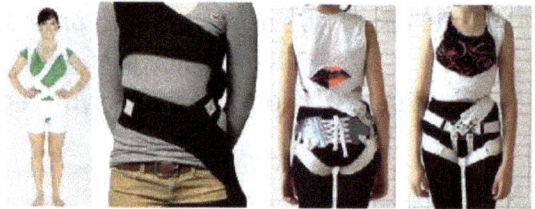

SpineCor brace (soft brace)

braces include the store-bought braces that may be found online and are sometimes called "posture correcting" braces. In no way are these a substitute for a custom-fitted brace and may cause a spine to become more "flat" in the upper back by pulling the shoulders back. For many types of scoliosis, this would be the opposite of what is needed.

- Nighttime Braces: The nighttime brace or "bending brace," is usually used for a single curve and does not correct in a 3 dimensional way (all planes of front, back, side to side and rotation). These braces, such as the Providence or Charleston brace, are made with the principle of "over-correcting" the curve. They fit very high under a person's arm, which pushes him/her

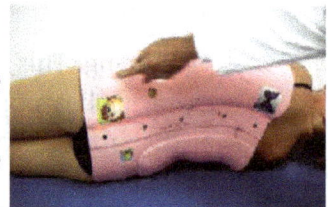

Nighttime Bending Brace

too far over to stand up and can be worn only at night. Interestingly, the human growth hormone in children has been shown to peak at night, so nighttime brace wearing is very helpful in correction regardless of brace type. Compliance may also be better at night since the nighttime brace doesn't interfere with a child's daytime activities. According to studies, full-time bracing treatment is necessary for a successful result as opposed to nighttime bracing only.

There are Different Types of Asymmetrical Braces
In studies, asymmetrical braces, in general, fared better than symmetrical or flexible braces in the correction of curvatures, providing more than 60% correction. A brace needs to be asymmetrical to push the spine into a corrective position in all three dimensions:

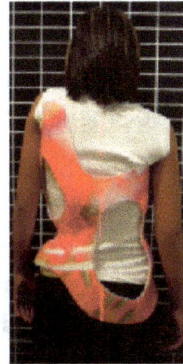

- Front - back

- Side - side

- and rotational planes.

- Also important is room for the concavity to expand away from the curve. As you can see in the following asymmetrical brace photos there is room for movement and room for breathing. The asymmetrical brace will not compress the spine, ribs and body evenly everywhere. The large curve correction made in these types of braces may partly compensate for the usual low compliance in the wearing of the brace.

Here are some examples of asymmetrical braces:

- Chêneau Type Brace: The original version succeeded in correcting the scoliosis curves, but regularly led to the formation of a "flat back" which is a problem with sagittal curves. Newer versions provide correction of all 3 planes and are much improved and avoid the flat back syndrome.

Chêneau Gensingen Brace by Dr Weiss®. The open spaces or "blowouts" within the brace leave room for the curved spine to move into a correction, leave room for breathing, and allow the muscles to receive less pressure in the weak areas, creating less muscle atrophy. This brace is lighter and smaller than most.

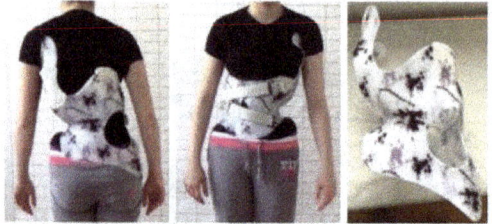
Gensingen brace (asymmetric brace)

- Rigo System Chêneau Brace: The Short RSC® Brace is the further development of the original Chêneau brace but follows a different curve classification system using Rigo curvature patterns (see curve classification discussion later in this chapter).

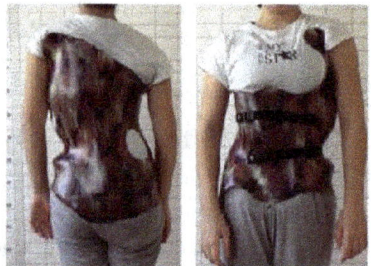
Rigo – Cheneau brace (rigid brace)

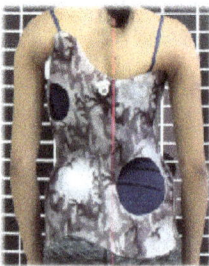
WCR Brace

- WCR (Wood Chêneau Rigo) Brace: Designed using the Rigo classification of scoliosis and brace design with some of the same principles as the Chêneau brace.

- The Whisper Brace. The Green Sun Medical Dynamic Brace (GSM) brace was developed as an alternative to rigid braces. The brace applies corrective forces while preserving range of motion. The brace components are prefabricated and adjusted for each patient. Modular components can be replaced to accommodate growth. A series of semi-rigid segments encircle the patient's torso and are joined by flexible (or elastic) elements to generate stabilizing forces, providing the necessary immobilization while allowing relative motion of the semi-rigid segments. To date, this brace is being tested to compare the curve correction to that of other braces.

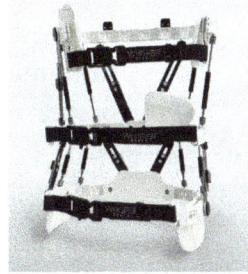

Whisper Brace

- The LA Brace™ is an asymmetrical brace based upon the Chêneau principles. The LA Brace uses a unique biomechanical classification system and is made with CAD/CAM technology. It is an asymmetrical design that strategically places pressure areas and void areas to maximize corrections. It is recommended to be worn day and night for the best outcome.

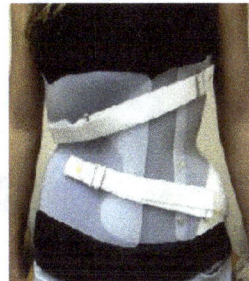

LA Brace

- PASB (Progressive Action Short Brace) is a custom-made thoraco-lumbar-sacral brace.

- ART Brace: The asymmetrical, rigid, torsion brace is constructed with 2 rigid asymmetrical pieces connected in the back at the midline by a bar. It has rigid ratcheting buckles and the upper third uses Velcro® straps.

- Milwaukee Brace: This cervical thoracic lumbar sacral brace has a pelvic girdle piece with metal uprights attached to a pad behind the head and a collar around the neck with a chin piece. Used from the 60s until the 80s. This brace has mostly gone out of use.

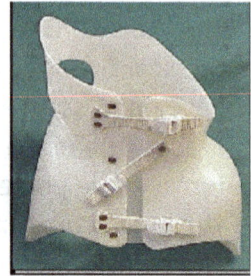

PASB Brace

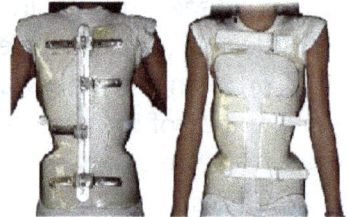

ART Brace

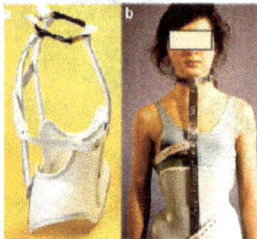

Milwaukee Brace

112

There are Different Types of Symmetrical Braces

- Boston Brace: In the early 70s, the most popular of the thoracic lumbar sacral braces, was the Boston Brace. It treats the coronal plane (side-to-side curves) and rotations of the thoracic, lumbar and sacral areas. This brace typically does not take into consideration the front-to-back sagittal curves. It can cause a flat back syndrome. This brace can either be prefabricated or custom-made.

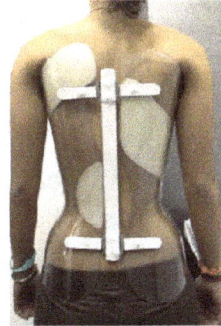

Boston Brace

- Dynamic Derotation Brace: A hard brace that reaches very high under the arms, it opens at the back and is equipped with specially designed bars to produce derotation. Braces that open in the back are much more difficult to get in and out of.

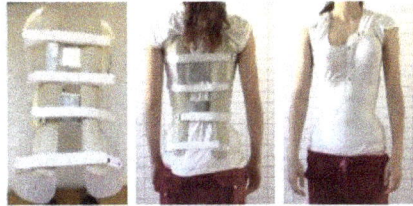

DDB brace (symmetric brace)

- Sforzesco Brace: Uses the SPoRT concept of bracing (Symmetrical, Patient-Oriented, Rigid, Three-dimensional)

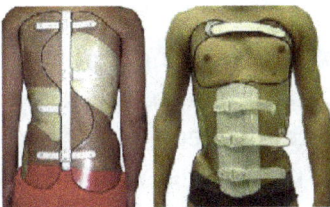

Sforzesco Brace

- The Lyon Brace: A thermoplastic rigid plastic brace with a bar in the back that has hinges to open and close the brace.

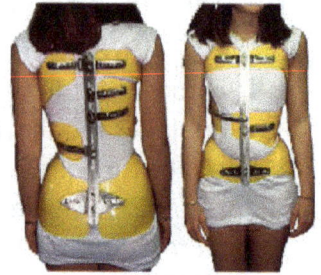

Lyon Brace

Do Your Research

You can see how different these braces can be. Making the best choice for your situation requires a bit of research on your part, but will be well worth the effort. Many doctors steer their patients toward a certain type of brace due to familiarity, preference, or a relationship with a specific brace facility. Perhaps your doctor may not have read the most recent research, as there are ever-evolving technologies. Your doctor may not have much faith in the process of bracing at all and discourage it. It is always the best plan of action to do your research before accepting an opinion or a referral without questioning. There are many types of braces and the referral may not be the best brace for you or your child. Do your research and interview orthotists in your area. It is an expensive and impactful tool in scoliosis care and the decision should not be a decision made lightly. There may be limited options where you live and travel may be needed to acquire the best brace for you and your situation. You likely won't need to visit the brace facility too often so the distance to a location shouldn't deter you.

While online information can be helpful for learning about different treatments for scoliosis, it is important to remember that every case of scoliosis is unique and may require a different approach. Only a professional medical practitioner with expertise in scoliosis can provide a proper diagnosis and develop a personalized treatment plan.

Cost of Brace and Treatment

When it comes to bracing, the average cost of a traditional scoliosis brace can vary depending on the design. Braces range in price from $3,000 to $10,000. It is important to ask if the price quoted is the total cost of the brace or if there are extra fees for having the brace fitted, X-rays taken, brace adjustments and any other associated fees. Sometimes two braces are offered, a day and a night brace, so that a more comfortable brace is worn during the day and a more corrective brace is worn at night. If a child is young, he or she is likely to outgrow the brace and need a new one at some point. Ask about this and the additional costs. Please see Chapter 17 "Resources," to find out about financial assistance.

Beware: There are numerous slick advertisements on the Internet for 1-3-week programs claiming to accomplish miraculous improvements in children's scoliosis. These "Boot Camp" programs are excessively priced and commonly require you to use their type of brace. **Please avoid these. Scoliosis NEVER responds to a "quick-fix" approach.**

What is an "In Brace Correction"?

When a brace is custom-made, an in-brace X-ray is usually taken within a few days to 6 weeks after fitting to determine how well the brace is correcting the curves. There is much debate about how much, or what percentage, of curve correction there must be for the brace to be considered effective. The amount of correction will be determined by the age of the patient, the stiffness of the spine, the size of the curve, the curve location and compliance with wearing the brace. A better curve correction in the brace indicates better success at the end of treatment. A minimum of 30% to 50% in-brace curve correction must be seen on X-ray before you can conclude that the brace is effective. Some practitioners like to mark the brace with a metal clip to show where the brace correction areas are so that it shows well on X-ray. This will guide the orthotist to make the best brace adjustments. These clips can be removed after the images are taken.

If the spine is still very flexible and/or the curve is between 20-30º it is not uncommon for a brace to over-correct and the spine curve may now look reversed on X-ray. This is a temporary condition and the spine will relax after brace weaning allowing the curve to settle back into a more neutral position.

Working With an Orthotist
When you first meet your orthotist for a consultation or to get started with making your brace, it might be an overwhelming experience for your child. The process will involve looking at the X-rays and doing an exam to take some very specific measurements of the torso. A digital scan might be taken of the torso to custom-create a brace. Always take notes at your appointments since a lot of information will be new and you will want to remember later. (At the end of this book I provide some interview question worksheets on page 245.)

When you are being evaluated, fitted and treated with your brace, communicate with your orthotist if your brace is hurting or causes sores. Tell your orthotist so it can be adjusted to make it more comfortable. Bring up any concerns that you have about wearing your brace. Your orthotist is part of your team and is here to help.

How is a Brace Made?

There are different terminologies for the practitioner fabricating the brace.

- Orthotist: The professional for the production and application of orthoses (Braces)
- CPO: Certified Orthotic and Prosthetic professional (American Board of Certification)

Once you have decided what type of brace is best for you or your child you should then research where the best facility is to have the brace measured and made. As recommended above, it may be worth traveling to find a good orthotist since it is likely that you won't have to visit too often. You need to work with somebody who has made hundreds of these braces and specializes in the art. If you live in a large city, there are probably many orthotists so you may be able to do some interviewing before deciding on such a large purchase that will impact your or your child's curvature and life. Once you have chosen your orthotist you will go for a consultation which may include reviewing the X-rays, an exam and discussing your goals. Measurements and photos may be made (measuring alone tends to have inconsistent results in fabricating a brace). Imaging, scanning, or casting may also be performed to get the best measurement for a brace.

What scanning/imaging or casting methods are used?

- CAD/CAM: Scanning (computer-aided design (CAD) and computer-aided manufacturing (CAM)). The patient is three-dimensionally scanned to create a topographical map of the entire torso, shoulders and pelvis. The digital scan as well as analysis of the images (X-ray or MRI etc.) are used to create a mold and then create a brace either by 3-D printing or by hand. Made out of plastic, the brace is lightweight and thin to increase compliance with wearing. Easily portable scanners mean that scanning can be performed in almost any location. Designs are easily repeatable. Electronic files are easily available and serve as documentation of a client's shape as changes happen over time. Not only can the design be made digitally, but testing its effectiveness and making modifications before actually fabricating and fitting it on a client can be done. Studies demonstrate significantly better in-brace correction with CAD/CAM compared to the traditional approach. It is also a faster process and without plaster casting, makes the experience much more comfortable.

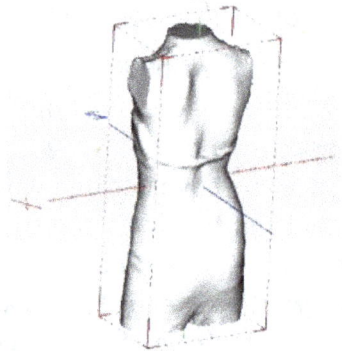

- Plaster Casting: Casting is the traditional method used to capture an impression of the body. The plaster cast method seems to be the most practiced technique for the construction of hard braces at the moment. The patient is fitted with a body stocking and then wet plaster is applied in sheets all around the torso while standing. Once it has dried this wrapping is cut away from the body and then used to make a mold of the torso. The mold is then shaved with a special tool to create a new shape. Plastic sheeting is then heated and applied by hand to this mold to create the brace. This is now shaped and molded to create the final brace.

Brace Fitting Protocol
From Ray Diaz, an orthotist in Los Angeles, who makes the Gensingen Cheneau brace: "The day I deliver the brace, I tighten the brace straps as snugly as possible and mark a line with a sharpie for the patient's reference. Two weeks later, I have them

118

return to prep them for in-brace X-rays. On this visit, I address whatever issues the patient may have. I re-tightened the straps and mark a new line for the patient's reference. The patient will then get the in-brace X-rays. Once the patient receives the X-ray, I have them send it to me for review. If the X-rays show less than a 30% reduction, I will have them return to me for adjustments. If there is a closer 40% to 50%, I will have them return in 3 months for a follow-up visit."

Follow Up X-rays?

Whether a person is in or out of a brace, follow-up imaging will be taken either to monitor a curve in the "watch and wait" scenario or to monitor the effectiveness of a brace. With a brace, there is no standard agreement as to when subsequent images should be taken and whether they are to be taken in or out of the brace. Each brace technician and orthopedist will have their own schedule and preference. Every 6 months is reasonable.

How long should the brace be off before taking a follow-up X-ray?

Out-of-brace images must be taken after the patient has spent some time not wearing the brace. There are many ways that each practitioner handles this scenario. One practitioner may want only in-brace imaging and forego the out-of-brace X-ray. Others may take an in-brace and out-of-brace X-ray on the same day (but then how will you know the true status of your curvature directly after directly taking off the brace?). Some practitioners will instruct you to take off your scoliosis brace for up to 24 hours before receiving an X-ray. This is not enough time to affect the treatment plan. Not all doctors are interested in an out-of-brace image until the end of brace treatment. Discuss your questions and concerns with your doctor to be sure you understand the instructions for these visits to avoid confusion or getting unnecessary X-rays.

Confused? It is best practice to take the brace off for 24 hours, before an out-of-brace X-ray, to allow full relaxation of the trunk to see the reliable status of the curve. You should always check with your orthotist and or your orthopedist to get out of brace X-ray instructions.

Soft braces are not recommended in the Schroth protocol. The Chêneau hard braces are highly recommended by Schroth practitioners. It is often worn 20–23 hours a day. Take it off to bathe and exercise only. For brace referrals check the SOSORT organization or website www.ScoliosisCoach.com

What is Curve Classification?
Another factor in brace creation is the classification of scoliosis. There are many methods used to classify a curve. The variations of scoliosis are endless, but some common patterns or classifications of scoliosis have been identified to determine bracing, surgery, or exercise therapy.

Curve classification methods:

- Cobb classification: John Robert Cobb invented it in 1948 to measure the curve angle between the top of the highest vertebra in the curve and the lowest. The Cobb angle, stated in degrees, measures the severity of the curve and is used to track changes over time.

- King classification is commonly used to analyze adolescent idiopathic scoliosis and vertebral fractures. It was first described in 1986 by Dr. James E. King, Jr.

- Lenke classification describes adolescent idiopathic scoliosis curvatures. Dr. Lawrence G. Lenke created it in 2001. This system analyzes spinal curve number, position and direction.

- Lehnert-Schroth classification describes scoliosis spinal curvatures. In the early 20th century, Christa Lehnert-Schroth and her mother, Katharina, devised it. It incorporates patient posture and spinal curvature location and orientation. This guides scoliosis exercise and physical therapy. The Lehnert-Schroth approach stresses muscular training, breathing and posture correction to treat scoliosis.

- SRS-Schwab classification describes curvatures in adults with spinal abnormalities such as scoliosis and kyphosis. SRS and Dr. Franz Schwab described it in the early 1990s. It evaluates the patient's age, skeletal maturity, spinal curvature magnitude and pattern and position and direction. This information helps choose surgical procedures and predict surgical outcomes.

- Roussouly classification determines high local stress zones in the whole spine. The lower the lumbar lordosis or flat back, the higher the stress is on the disks; the more the lumbar lordosis increases, the more the contact force on the posterior column.

- Barcelona Physical Therapy School (BSPTS) classification (illustrated next page) groups four scoliosis curve types. This guides scoliosis exercise and physical therapy.

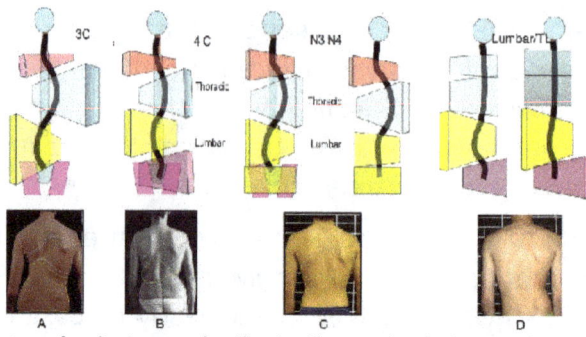

The BSPTS system of scoliosis curve classification illustrated with photographs and body block diagrams. The four scoliosis curve types in this classification system are 3C (a), 4C (b), N3N4 (c), and single lumbar or thoracolumbar (d). The 3C curve is a major thoracic scoliosis curve with a compensatory lumbar and pelvic shift (a). The 4C curve is a major lumbar scoliosis curve with a thoracic and lumbar shift (b). The N3N4 curve is a major thoracic scoliosis with or without a lumbar curve but with the pelvis in a neutral position (c). The single lumbar or thoracolumbar curve is a single curve scoliosis with an uncoupled pelvic shift and no thoracic curvature (d)

Bracing History

Bracing, or orthotic treatment of spinal disorders, dates back at least to the Middle Ages *ca* 400 *to* 1600 AD). Some of the concepts of those early bracing devices, notably three-point forces, are still used today. Fabrication materials have progressed from metal and leather to lightweight plastics allowing many new designs and a new level of comfort for the wearer.

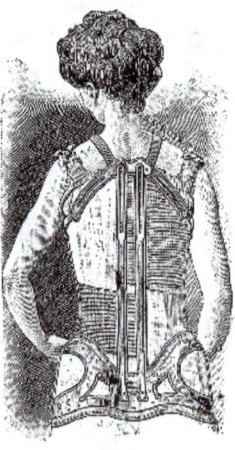

Vintage Scoliosis Brace

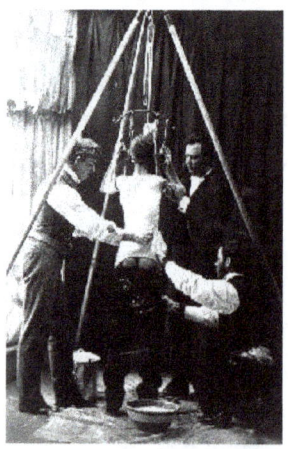

Vintage Plaster Casting

122

What determines the success of a brace?

The outcome of brace treatment depends on many factors:

- IBC: In Brace Correction, as discussed earlier, is defined as the percentage of curve reduction visualized on an X-ray while wearing the brace. Varying studies report that a 10-25% in-brace correction of the curve is needed for a successful outcome but no consensus has been reached on the exact percentage. A minimum of 30-50% in-brace correction is highly recommended in the industry regardless of the studies. Further research is necessary to establish the minimum in-brace correction rate that should be attained. In-brace correction imaging will show only a side-to-side correction of a curvature. A lateral (side view) is also essential to see if a correction has been made in the front-to-back curvatures of the spine. "Flat-back" can result if a brace is improperly made and the low back (inward curve) and upper back (outward curve) must be supported/corrected for scoliosis correction to be successful.

- Compliance: The better a person complies with wearing his or her brace, the better the outcome. Research has variable conclusions regarding the minimum hours required to be successful but all research agrees that compliance is the key to success. Some orthotists will provide a monitoring system such as the iButton Thermal Sensor. This sensor is dime-sized and records the internal temperature of the brace to track how much it is worn. Always strive to wear the brace for as many hours as your orthotist suggests. I will discuss exact brace-wearing times later in this chapter. Team management is crucial to increase compliance. Your team may consist of an orthopedic surgeon, orthotist, physiotherapist, chiropractor, Schroth practitioner, psychologist, massage therapist and support group(s). Some studies confirm that a team approach increased quality of life scores, compliance and success by up to 5 times!

Brace Wear Time Vs. Effectiveness

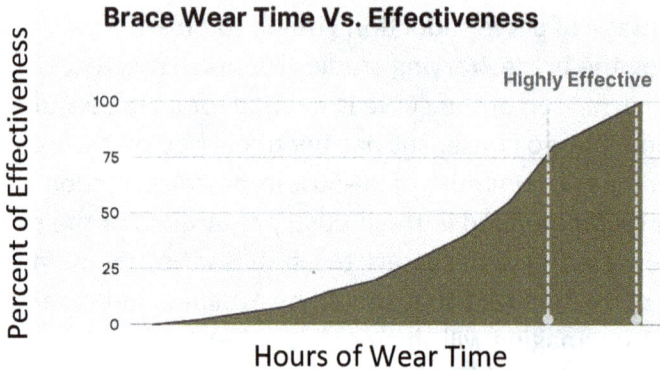

Highly Effective

Y-axis: Percent of Effectiveness (100, 75, 50, 25, 0)

X-axis: Hours of Wear Time

- Brace Tightness: The term "quality of bracing" was first introduced by Lou, *et al.* (2004) and has been used to describe the tightness of a brace. Researchers have found a positive correlation between tightness and treatment outcomes. However, the method of tightening the brace and the degree of tightness depends on the orthotist's expertise. I have had some patients who over-tightened the brace and caused pressure sores and others who wore it too loosely or wore an ill-fitting brace too long before getting it adjusted or remade. Follow your orthotist's guidance but don't be afraid to speak up if something doesn't feel right! If you are having trouble tightening your straps try lying down or leaning against a wall to get better leverage or ask a friend or family member to help.

- Growth Stage: Most physicians recommend starting a brace or weaning out of a brace based purely on a person's age, growth stage (bone maturity), voice change, or menstruation status. This is called a Growth Classification and there are a few ways to do this. Studies have shown the variable significance of a person's growth status on the bracing

124

outcome. The late growth stages (Risser 4, etc.) are sometimes used to discourage the use of a brace as being "too late" but it is the author's opinion (and research supports it) that it can be a mistake to miss an opportunity to correct or stabilize a curve, as small growth is still a possibility and the spine is possibly still flexible. Please see the "Research" chapter 21 to learn more about studies on scoliosis treatment past the skeletal maturity markers.

There are various growth classification systems that your physician may use:

- Sanders, Greulich-Pyle, Tanner-Whitehouse and the Thumb Ossification Composite Index (TOCI) methods are based on an X-ray of the left hand and the state of ossification ("sealing" of the growth plates) of the bones.

- Risser Sign is based on an X-ray of pelvic bones.

Outgrowing the Brace
Typically, if a child has grown 2 inches since the brace was fitted it is time for a new brace. It will no longer be pressurizing the correct areas. Girls may develop breasts or hip bones that no longer fit well into a brace and a new brace or brace adjustment may need to be made even if they haven't grown the 2".

Brace Weaning Off Phase
General guidelines: The Society on Scoliosis Orthopedic and Rehabilitation Treatment (SOSORT) proposed that the brace weaning-off phase should initiate at 75% growth stage (or Risser 4). It is also widely recommended that weaning should begin at either 15 or 16 years of age or as soon as girls menstruate, or 17 years of age, or the cracking of the voice for boys. For larger curves weaning may be delayed even further.

Other Schools of Thought: It is widely thought that bracing after skeletal maturity is useless, even if some studies show that curve correction can continue or curve progression can be prevented if the use of the brace is sustained past this initial period. A child can grow for as many as two years after the growth plates have closed on an X-ray. The conclusion of a study by Negrini, Atanasio and Fusco in 2009 revealed that before the age of 20, even in skeletally mature people, it is possible to reach more curve improvement both visually and by X-ray, although not as significantly as during growth. Skeletal maturity or the onset of menstruation may not always be the best indicator for early or rapid weaning out of a brace. Brace correction is based on bone growth, but ligaments and neuromuscular control of posture can also be involved. If a person is possibly still growing or the skeleton is still maturing or is still quite flexible, bracing should continue for a while past Risser 4 or menstruation.

How long should weaning off a brace take? For a typical full-time brace, it is advisable to reduce the brace-wearing time by a couple of hours per day for a few months and then possibly wear the brace only at night for up to another six months. Your orthotist will have a plan so be sure to ask questions and stick to the schedule. It is this author's opinion that after a stressful battle of bracing, therapy, cost and effort, it is a shame to stop treatment too early and possibly lose ground. Stay the course as long as possible. Talk to your doctor and orthotist and if pressured to stop, ask why and for any possible downside to wearing the brace a bit longer, unless of course, the patient has outgrown the brace! If you compare a scoliosis brace to orthodontics on the teeth, no one would take the braces off the teeth until directed and 6 months later expect the teeth to have stayed straight without a retainer. Teeth would be unable to hold their new position because ligaments are still too long on one side of the tooth and too short on the other side. The imbalance in the tension would

126

pull on the tooth until it returned to its previously crooked position. The retainer for the teeth or the brace for the spine has to be worn 24 hours per day, then time is reduced until the patient is wearing it only at night. Many patients continue to wear their retainer at night into early adulthood to ensure tooth alignment is not lost. Why should we treat the alignment of the spine any differently than the alignment of teeth?

If anything, spinal alignment is more complicated and unstable than a tooth. When a patient is ready to reduce time in the scoliosis brace, the doctor or orthotist may instruct the patient to remain out-of-brace for progressively longer periods before taking a standing image. The weaning process for nighttime scoliosis bracing typically involves gradually reducing the amount of time that the brace is worn each night, under the supervision of a doctor or orthotist. The goal of the weaning process is to allow the patient's spine to gradually adjust to the changes that have occurred during treatment and to minimize the risk of relapse.

After brace weaning: At or after brace weaning, some loss of correction is expected in 30% to 43% of people, mostly in the first 6 months. Early weaning may lead to greater curve progression rates and regular curve monitoring should be done every 4–6 months until skeletal maturity. Scoliosis-specific postural exercises can markedly reduce the loss of correction at brace weaning, so the implementation of exercises at that stage could potentially stabilize curve progression.

Flat Back Syndrome
The spine has natural curves in the sagittal or front-to-back direction that act as a spring or shock absorber. These curves are critical to the health of the spine but can become problematic in many scoliosis cases. The curves can become flat or overly curved and must be addressed as part of the treatment of scoliosis to

have the best outcome. Some braces do not take these natural curves into account and in some cases, can actually flatten these curves. This "flat back syndrome" also occurs in some scoliosis fusion surgeries. It is important to discuss these curves when making a treatment plan with any physical therapist or orthotist (bracing) professional. Ignoring these important curves will impair the success of a scoliosis correction.

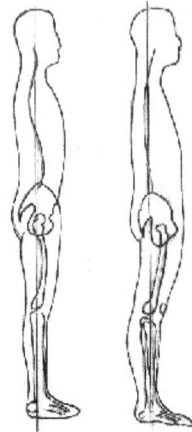

Normal alignment VS. Flat Back

Adult Bracing

Adult curves can progress as much as a degree or more per year if left untreated. Based on studies by the Scoliosis Research Society, there is strong evidence to support the use of brace treatment for adult idiopathic (unknown cause) scoliosis due to reported short-term improvement in pain and curve stabilization. For curves at high risk of progression, rigid and daytime braces are recommended. There is an increasing interest in adult bracing and in my personal experience, it has been rewarding for my adult patients. The other benefit to adult bracing is that it is usually possible to wear the brace on an "as needed" basis and also for substantially fewer hours per day than a child is required to wear. Usually, these braces are very low profile supporting only the lower spine, sometimes called a short brace. My patients have reported that they felt much more secure and comfortable as well as had a reduction in their pain when wearing a short brace. The other good news is that the brace won't get outgrown. The role of scoliosis posture-specific exercise such as Schroth, in combination with bracing, still needs to be studied in adults, but there is good evidence so far that bracing results can be enhanced with scoliosis-specific exercise. People with degenerative scoliosis with rotatory dislocation and disc instability could also potentially become good candidates for a short brace.

How Many Hours Does Your Brace Need to Be Worn?
The prescribed wearing time is directly related to the Cobb angle (degrees of the curve) and will vary based on your case and your orthotist. Usually, when you first begin wearing a brace you will ease into it with possibly a few hours a day, increasing daily. But every orthotist and every patient is different. Typically, these are the following wearing times for a full-time brace, not a nighttime brace.

Full-time for curves over 40° is 22 hours
Full-time for curves between 35-40° is 20–24 hours
Part-time for curves between 30-34° is 16-24 hours
Part-time for curves between 25-29° is 12-24 hours

Night-time bracing typically will be 8 hours for curves less than 25°.

As discussed earlier, compliance is critical to the success of a brace and reducing curvature. Wearing a brace full-time is associated with a much lower surgical rate than wearing the brace part-time. The brace should be taken off to bathe and in addition to any scoliosis-specific exercises or physical therapy. Sports also make it difficult to wear a brace. Some take it off or loosen it to eat.

What to Wear Under a Brace?

A shirt should be worn under the brace and next to the skin but the options are endless! Wear something comfortable because the brace will be on your body for many hours. An undershirt will improve comfort and reduce the risk of skin abrasions and sweat rashes.

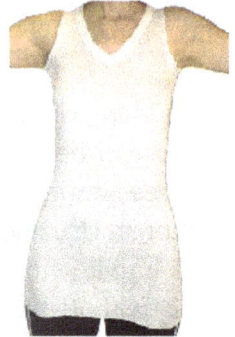

Anything under a scoliosis brace needs to be:

- Ideally be cotton or bamboo and possibly a material that is anti-bacterial, moisture-wicking and anti-microbial. Nylon or polyester gets hot and sticky and sore areas of the skin could develop.

- Tight fitting: If it is too large or has wrinkles you will experience chafing and rubbing.

- Seamless, or wear the shirt inside out.

- Thick enough to provide skin protection and not get ruined by the brace.

- Thin enough to not be too hot.

- Long enough to run the length of the brace.

- High enough in the armpits to provide protection or even a "flap" over the armpit.

- http://scoliosisliving.blogspot.com/2014/04/what-to-wear-under-your-scoliosis-brace.html

Here are some great vendors/sites to shop:

- The Scoliosis Tank on Etsy has a flap to cover brace edges under the arm.

- scokhloetees@gmail.com for a custom order of t-shirts that offer a little padding in the armpit area for your brace type.

130

- Brace Buddies
- Hope's Closet at Align Clinic
- SO Seamless Tanks (Kohls)
- Sanaa's ScoKhloeTees for WCR Braces
- www.Tillys.com Torso "Sock" – with or without flap to protect against brace edges
- http://royalknit.com/products/torso-socks/
- http://www.bostonbrace.com/content/accessories.asp
- Sugar Lips (No underarm flap)
- SmartKnitKIDS Seamless or compression
- Uniqlo
- EmBraced in Comfort
- Singlosport
- DiabeticSock
- The Boston T (with armpit flap) is a protective body sock made of CoolMAX/Lycra, with an antibacterial fiber
- BraceBuddies
- Rosette seamless shirts
- Under Amour™ seamless shirts
- For Boys: Jockey Seam-Free Crew, Fun and Function Tees, Sierra Trading Post T-shirt

The seams and bands of elastic on some bras and underwear can be too thick, irritating the skin. Smoother seamless underwear will be more comfortable. Sports-style bras work best because of their softness and comfort and there is no clasp in the back. Finding one with bands that aren't too thick or wide will help under the brace. Some are more comfortable with a "bralet" for a more sleek or lower profile.

What to Wear Over a Brace?
Usually, clothes 1 or 2 sizes larger are required. Here is a typical shopping list from our brace-wearing friends.

- Shorts
- Tanks
- Thin long sweater: with most braces extending 3/4 of the way down the hips and glutes, a long sweater can cover well.
- Loose t-shirts
- Kimonos
- Lightweight long sleeves, or 3/4 length and layers are always good.
- Patterns hide the brace lines in the front and back. Shirts that hang down past the hips hide any brace lines on the pants.
- A camisole worn over the brace can protect clothing from the velcro straps and give the layered look.
- Elastic-waisted jeans or lycra leggings prevent bulky seams and can be worn over or under the brace.
- Long skirts and miniskirts with elastic waists.
- Shoulder pad on one side to make shoulders appear more even due to the lifted axillary extension in some braces.
- https://www.bracingforscoliosus.org/what-to-wear-what-not-to-wear/
- https://nationalscoliosiscenter.com/topics/fashion/
- https://scoliosis3dc.com/2018/07/09/what-to-wear-with-scoliosis/ https://scoliosis3dc.com/2018/04/06/best-shirt-to-wear-under-a-scoliosis-brace/

Sleeping in a Brace

It will take some time to adjust to sleeping with a brace, considering it is usually made of hard, inflexible material. Many have indicated that they got used to it fairly quickly (within days or weeks). If the brace is cutting into you, talk to the orthotist who may add some extra foam in certain areas (along the back edge for example) and shave down some areas a bit. Talk to your orthotist about wearing it a bit loosely at night. This allows for some movement to find a more comfortable position; then you can gradually tighten it to the tension that was recommended by the orthotist. Using a pillow assortment and adding a mattress topper for extra padding may be helpful. It is very important to find a way to make sleep as comfortable as possible since a lack of sleep will have a detrimental impact on daily life and can reduce compliance.

Side sleeping with a pillow between your knees and under the top arm can be very comfortable and supportive.

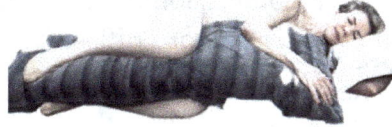

I use a body pillow and cannot sleep without it! Sleeping on your back can give your curves the best support and requires no extra pillows except maybe under your knees. As we saw in Chapter 9 "Bracing," the human growth hormone in children has been shown to peak at night, so nighttime brace wearing is very helpful in correction regardless of brace type. Compliance may also be better at night since the nighttime brace doesn't interfere with a child's daytime activities. According to studies, full-time bracing treatment is necessary for a successful result as opposed to nighttime bracing only. We will take about mattresses later.

What Problems Can Develop With Bracing?

There are some possible adverse consequences of bracing:

- Pain

- Nausea
- Tingling
- Skin irritation
- Kidney disorders
- Psychosocial issues
- Difficulty breathing
- Difficulty eating large meals - eat small meals more often as a remedy.
- Weight loss due to eating discomfort

Braces are designed to fit tightly against the body and that can lead to skin irritation from heat or rubbing. Protecting the skin is important. Always wear a thin, tight-fitting, sweat-wicking shirt under the brace. Some redness is normal when wearing a brace, but call your doctor's office if:

- Redness doesn't go away within 30 minutes after taking off the brace.
- Blisters or sores develop.
- A rash appears on the skin under the brace.

It is very important not to self-treat any skin irritation without discussing it with your orthotist or doctor. Some remedies may make the skin more susceptible to irritation. Cortisone-type creams for example, actually cause the skin to become softer, thinner and delicate, which makes it more susceptible to irritation. Some of my patients have used adhesive silicone gel bandages such as Hydro Seal®, to protect any sore areas of the skin. Please always ask your orthotist about this before using it. Ask your orthotist if baby powder or cornstarch on your skin is a good idea. In my clinic, I have tried moleskin on any areas of the brace that have rough spots, edges, or rivets. Be cautious with lotions or oils on the skin under the brace as they can cause skin irritation.

What If My Child Won't Wear It?
Most kids do well with wearing their brace. But when children struggle, an understanding parent can make a big difference. You can make the day-to-day reality of wearing a brace easier just by being there for your child as a supporter and cheerleader. Encourage your child to come to you when things get tough. Promise you will listen. Don't jump in with solutions unless you are asked for your help. Then, work together to come up with solutions and incentives to get your child to wear the brace. Agree on the occasional "night off" for important events, like a dance or beach day. Discuss with your orthotist any modification that you make to the schedule, including sports, etc. Your care team is a resource for you and your child. Your care team knows that some kids struggle with wearing a brace at times and can give you tips and ideas on how to handle the challenge. The internet is a great resource to reach out to and find support groups. Facebook and Instagram have many groups for all different types of discussion topics. Read Chapter 16 "Psychology" and 17 "Resources" for a robust list of great ideas to help your child along.

Finding a scoli-buddy or two can be a life-changing support network even if it is only virtual. The odds that there are others with scoliosis in your immediate circle are good. If you just reach out and ask you will be surprised to find a scoli-buddy with which to share your journey. Some parents have come up with a reward system for wearing the brace and it seems to work. This is your parenting choice!

Taking Care of the Brace

Follow the instructions from your provider for cleaning and caring for the brace. Clients have said using a baby wipe is the best way to clean a brace but always ask your orthotist. If any part of your brace should break it is important to have that fixed only by the orthotist who created it if possible. Never modify the brace yourself. Some clients carry their brace in a large bag and have fun with the design. Having fun with the brace, declaring it a "coat of armor" or flipping the attitude about it in any way can prove helpful. Why not decorate it? Try out some ideas on plastic containers first to see what might or might not work. Decoupage, tapes, sharpies, stickers, or rub-ons can be fun and are easy to replace as desired. Sometimes I discover that there is a rough spot of plastic on the inside of the brace from manufacturing and it is easily rubbed down with a nail file or light sandpaper. If having the brace at school is a problem (small lockers, etc.) ask a school nurse or P.E. teacher to safely store it. A note for school is sometimes needed for any special circumstances regarding gym/P.E. exemptions or sitting at a desk.

Recycling a brace
Some people keep the brace after outgrowing it and others wonder what to do with the brace. It is a custom-made medical product but it can be repurposed!
Embrace Foundation was founded in 2018 to accept donations and repurpose used DME (Durable Medical Equipment) for under-served people around the world. All items collected are distributed through Samaritan's Purse® World Medical Mission.
https://www.embrace-foundation.org/what-we-do/
FOCOS A non-profit organization with a mission to provide access to optimum orthopedic care to improve the quality of life in Ghana and other countries.
https://focos.focoshospital.org/our-story/

Other Types of Braces:

The physio-logic® brace by Dr. Weiss to improve sagittal curves of lumbar "flat back".

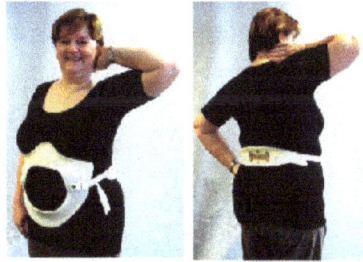

The Kyphologic brace® 2005:
A design for kyphosis by Dr. Weiss, to improve sagittal curves of thoracic kyphosis, a convex curvature "round back".

The Spondylogic® 2005 by Dr. Weiss.
A brace designed for spinal instabilities such as spondylolisthesis (Anterior lumbar vertebrae displacement).

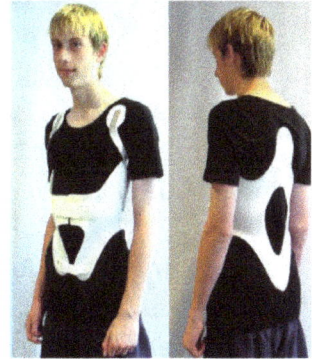

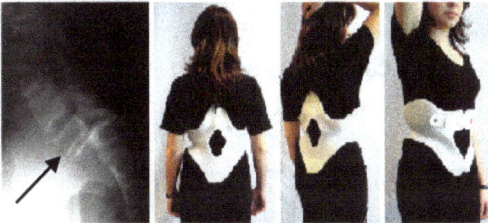

Spondylolisthesis

What Does the Research Show?

- There is strong evidence for bracing in idiopathic (unknown cause) scoliosis.

- Some braces are better than others.

- There has been an apparent improvement in the effectiveness of bracing in reducing surgical rates since 2005, related to the types of brace.

- For curves at high risk of progression, rigid and full-time braces are recommended.

- Scoliosis-specific postural exercises (such as Schroth) as a supplement to bracing can further improve the treatment result.

- Day-Time vs. Night-Time Brace: Katz et al. (1997) showed that the Boston brace (day) was more effective than Charleston (night) brace in avoiding progression. Their findings were most notable for curves initially between 36-45º. 83% of Charleston and 43% of Boston groups progressed. According to the authors, Charleston could be useful only in mild curves. Howard et al. (1998) compared the TLSO with the Charleston and Milwaukee braces and found that the TLSO was superior to both at preventing curve progression.

Comparing Brace Concepts

There are multiple types of braces and the research is interesting. Please read Chapter 21 "Research" for more details. From the data, it is apparent that asymmetrical braces are more effective than symmetrical braces with ARTbrace and Chêneau Gensingen braces ranking high in correction.

Bracing Combined with Scoliosis Specific Exercise

Rigo et al. (2003) in a study with 106 subjects used the Chêneau brace with Schroth exercises and achieved a 94.4% of success rate in terms of avoiding surgery.

Negrini et al. (2008) combined bracing with SEAS (Scientific Exercises Approach to Scoliosis) exercises getting a success rate of 95.5%, but the mean curve (Cobb) angle was very low (23.4º), so patients with a low risk of progression were included.

A study on the conservative approach, with brace and exercises, was made in 2009 and reported only 4% of progression. All curve patterns improved, except for the double major type.

Videos About Braces

https://www.youtube.com/@socalscoliosiscare/featured
https://youtu.be/GkKPNIksFmg
https://youtu.be/3cxSqsdKo3g

10. WILL IT GET WORSE?

There are many factors to determine if a curve can get better or may get worse.

- Gender: Although both boys and girls develop mild scoliosis at about the same rate, girls have a much higher risk of the curve worsening and requiring treatment.

- Spinal flexibility

- Compliance with brace: see Chapter 9 "Bracing"

- Compliance with scoliosis-specific postural exercises and daily habits/posture correction

- Size of the curve: larger curves have a greater risk of progression. In patients with severe thoracic curves (greater than 90-100°), there is an increased risk of lung and heart issues. However, an increased death rate has not been found in long-term studies of patients with idiopathic scoliosis.

- If the curves are balanced or unbalanced: Larger and more unbalanced curves (one large and one small) tend to increase over time. Prognosis is best when the curves are symmetrical.

- Family history: Scoliosis can run in families. There is great interest in DNA-based tests to determine who is at risk of developing scoliosis and which patients with scoliosis are most likely to progress. However, the current understanding of the relationship between genetic factors and environmental factors in the development of scoliosis remains limited.

- Age: Signs and symptoms typically begin in adolescence and can progress rapidly during this time.

- Smaller curves tend to stay stable and in some cases, may correct themselves as the child grows.

- Curve progression before skeletal maturity occurs in approximately two-thirds of cases and in 10% of patients, it progresses to severe scoliosis (Cobb angle greater than 40°) in the following years.

- Potential for growth: Height measured over time that shows no change over a few months is a sure sign growth is slowing or done. X-rays of the pelvic bone (Risser) or of the hand may also show the growth plates. Breast development and first period in girls, voice change and facial hair in boys also indicate skeletal maturity status.

Age and Curve Size: Progression
A scientific study published in Spine observed over 200 children with scoliosis and followed the progression of their scoliosis.

Cobb Angle Rapid Change

During the critical period between 11 to 14 years old, curves can grow rapidly. Watching and waiting during this period can result in loss of valuable treatment time.

Critical Period

11-14 years of age = critical period

■ Curve Degrees

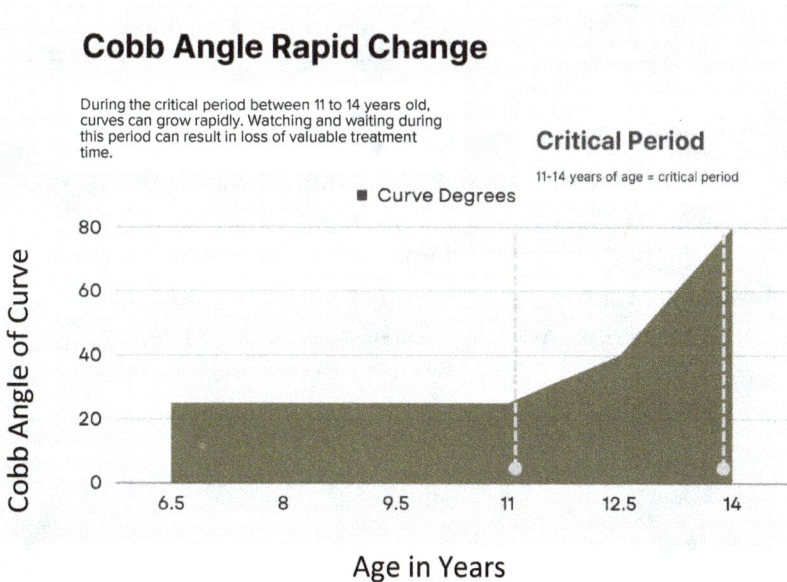

Cobb Angle of Curve (y-axis): 0, 20, 40, 60, 80

Age in Years (x-axis): 6.5, 8, 9.5, 11, 12.5, 14

Once a teen reaches skeletal maturity the risk of a curve increasing drops significantly but some studies have shown not to take your eye off it too quickly. Studies show that continued brace and therapy after skeletal maturity can continue to help the curve reduce and remain stable longer.

The risk for progression in the following chart is adapted from the study by Nachemson *et al.* describing the progression rate for children ten to sixteen years old with curves of various sizes.

Curve Size/Degrees	Age and Associated Progression Rate	Age and Associated Progression Rate	Age and Associated Progression Rate
	10-12 Years Old	13-15 Years Old	16 Years Old
19º or less	25%	10%	0%
20-29º	60%	40%	10%
30-39º	90%	70%	30%
60º	100%	90%	70%

You can see in the table above that both the size of the curve, as well as age, are directly related to the rate of progression. The younger the patient and the larger the curve, the more likely scoliosis will progress. Nachemson *et al.* also found that bracing was 40% more effective than observation only in preventing progression of more than 6º; despite the poorly fit braces of the time (1995).

Looking at the table below adapted from a study by Lonstein *et al.* we again see that as the child progresses to skeletal maturity, the less likely their scoliosis is to progress and that progression is also linked to the size of the initial curve as well as the age of the child.

Percentage Chance of Scoliosis Progression Based on Curve Size and Age at First Exam

Age First Examined	5-19º Curve Size/Degrees	20-29º Curve Size/Degrees
10 and younger	45%	100%
11-12	23%	61%
13-14	8%	37%
15 and older	4%	16%

Again, the argument against the "watch and wait method" is illustrated here by the high risk of curve progression.

Which respect to adults, studies of patients with adolescent idiopathic scoliosis after skeletal maturity, found that curves less than 30° do not progress, while most curves greater than 50° continue to progress. Adults can progress as much as a degree or more per year if left untreated.

Other Scoliosis Facts:

- As the thoracic spine is more rigid due to the ribs, the percentage of correction achieved through bracing is less than that of the thoracolumbar and lumbar spine.
- Moderate curves correct less with bracing when compared with milder curves.
- Some curve patterns are easier or more difficult to correct.
- Some individuals have a very strong curve or a very stiff spine, making correction difficult.

143

- Very large curves may be difficult to correct but this in no way indicates that it is not worth attaining as much correction as possible.

- BMI (Body Mass Index) is used to determine if an adolescent is underweight, normal weight, or overweight (greater than the 84th percentile). People with both high and low BMI have a greater risk for brace failure.

- Type of Brace: Rigid vs. soft braces. (See Chapter 21 "Research")

- Day-time vs. night-time brace: Studies show that Boston and TLSO braces perform better than night-time only braces.

- Rotation of the spine, for example, can affect the appearance and progression of the curve and it's important for physicians to accurately measure and track the amount of rotation present.

- Osteopenia, or low bone density, can also impact the effectiveness of certain treatments, such as spinal fusion surgery.

- The presence of the ERα and TPH-1 genes has been linked to an increased risk of developing scoliosis, which may also affect how the condition progresses.

- The speed at which the curve corrects over time is another important factor, as a slow correction rate may indicate that the curve is unlikely to stabilize without intervention.

11. WHAT SHOULD I AVOID?

Studies have ruled out the idea that adolescent idiopathic scoliosis curves are caused by specific behaviors such as regularly carrying heavy loads or "bad posture", but that does not mean that these factors do not have any impact on scoliosis. Knowing what NOT to do might be as important as knowing what the best treatment is for scoliosis. Avoiding things that can irritate or worsen a curve can also help with pain relief. As we know, all of the curves of the spine must be considered with scoliosis. In our daily lives, we may be encouraging scoliosis (or other curve disturbances) to become worse if we are chronically moving into an undesirable posture or exercise.

Sports
High-impact sports such as gymnastics, basketball, running, track, etc., are possibly detrimental to scoliosis as the spine absorbs much of the impact and can irritate sagittal and scoliosis curves (front-to-back as well as side-to-side curves). The spine is a natural shock absorber when it is healthy and has ideal sagittal curves. When these curves are disrupted, the shock absorption ability is compromised. Also, highly competitive sports (professional-level exertion) can release hormones in growing children that are detrimental to scoliosis.

Side Bending Sports/Exercises

Just about every scoliosis has a curve that
creates an "S" or a "C" shape. This lateral bend
of the spine typically exhibits a "strong side"
and a "weak side". When performing a side
bend exercise, the curve may be made worse
(bending into the concavity). But if the curve is
bent in the opposite direction it may be
stretching the weak muscles on the concave
side of the curve. The spine is likely to have
one, two, or even three lateral scoliosis curves.
The muscles inside the concavity of these curves are
fundamentally weak and do not need to be stretched with a
lateral bend "away from the curve." Lateral bending to
"straighten a curve" is also very likely to bend other curves even
worse into their concavity! Lateral bending should be avoided as a
repetitive movement or as a remedy for scoliosis.

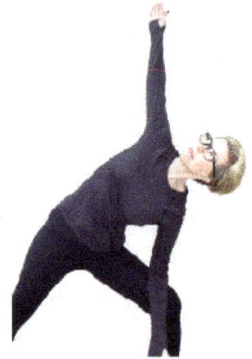

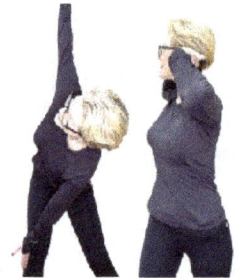

Rotating Sports/Exercises

Just about every curve has a rational
component in the spine possibly in multiple
areas going in different directions. Repetitive
rotating can irritate an already rotated spine
and it is difficult to isolate rotation to one area
or be sure what direction is best for you.
Rotation should be avoided as a repetitive
movement or as a remedy for scoliosis.

Front to Back (Sagittal) Sports/Exercises

Very commonly people with scoliosis will have a
disturbance in the natural sagittal curves of the
spine (the front-to-back curves). The curves can become flattened
or exaggerated meaning the inward or outward curves are not
quite where they belong, they may be too high or too low, too big

(kyphosis), or too flat (flat back) this leads us to a discussion on flat back syndrome.

Flat Back Syndrome

Very commonly those with scoliosis will have a "flat back" meaning a loss of the thoracic kyphosis (outward curve of the upper back). If this is you, then you need to be aware of what movements can make this worse. Upper back extension (back bend) will only encourage the area to be flat. This could be as simple as resting or sleeping on your belly, bending backward over a foam roller or a chair to stretch or "crack" your back. Some exercises will also cause you to arch your upper back resulting in more flattening of the area. Be aware of your habits and make the needed changes. In this case, you will need to encourage kyphosis (roundness) in the upper back/thoracic spine if you have a flattening of the area, unless contraindicated (if for example, you have osteoporosis). If you have any questions you should check with your physical therapist or Schroth practitioner for ideas on how to improve a flat back syndrome.

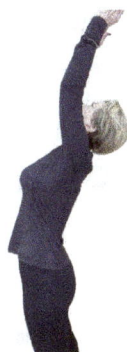

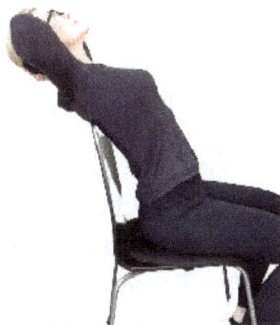

When attempting to fix a flat back, we should assume that the patient needs to "round" the area, working into thoracic rounding. The concern is that forward rounding makes scoliosis look worse. However one must realize that we are looking at two different things - the spine flatness vs. the rib rotation causing a "bump". The concern is that focusing on rounding will make the "bump" worse, but we need to focus on the SPINE into improved rounding and not look at the rib "bump". Likewise, if the flatness is in the lower spine then we need to encourage the inward arch in the lumbar spine. Though they cannot cause the condition, activities that involve deep backbends and spinal position alteration may lead to scoliotic curve progression. I am not saying that you cannot do these certain tasks, just that you should be aware that they may affect your overall condition in the future.

Kyphosis
Causes of kyphosis:

- Postural dysfunction
- Scheuermann's Disease
- Congenital kyphosis
- Kyphosis secondary to trauma
- Tumors
- Infection
- Arthritis

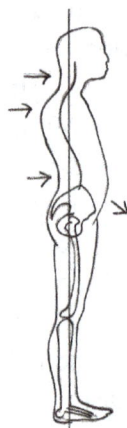

Kyphosis is classified as either postural or structural. Postural is attributed to poor postural habits leading to core and trunk weakness. Structural kyphosis is caused by an abnormality affecting the bones, discs, or muscles. Kyphosis with a structural cause may require medical intervention because the patient alone cannot control curve progression. Abnormal kyphotic curves are usually found in the thoracic or thoracolumbar spine but can be cervical. Kyphotic posture may present as a jutting chin, tight chest, posterior neck muscles, weak muscles of the spine and backward tilted pelvis and in extreme cases, respiration may be inhibited. This postural condition can be addressed using scoliosis-specific postural exercises and breathing exercises with proper instruction, postural re-education and consistent healthy lifestyle choices. Early treatment is important to control curve progression, especially with adolescents. I avoid the terms "Hunchback or Dowagers Hump" as they are negative triggering

148

descriptions and our goal is to be encouraging and positive when referring to a person's spine. Yes, you can get braced, even for kyphosis. See Chapter 9 "Bracing".

Dos and Don'ts with Kyphosis & Scoliosis:

- Avoid texting with the head down. The neck bends forward when we text. This harms the natural neck curve and applies pressure on the spinal cord. (See chapters 7 & 12 for remedies)

- Do not lift heavy objects. Carrying heavy things compresses your spine and it often does so asymmetrically. This applies to those with scoliosis as well.

- Avoid belly sleeping. The spine usually twists and the hips rotate to get truly comfortable and this may not be beneficial to your spine. Ask your Schroth therapist for sleeping posture guidance. This photo is an example of how belly sleeping crates multiple zones of rotations.

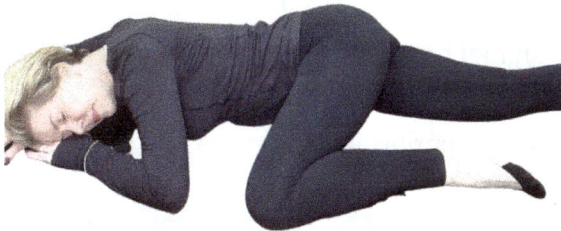

- Housework: With scoliosis, there will be a dominant side of muscle strength (and a weaker side) and when doing housework, etc., I suggest using the less dominant side. Ask your Schroth therapist if you need postural guidance.

- School/Work Ergonomics: Sitting and shifting the wrong way at your desk can put pressure on the curve and on the already dominant side. Crossing the legs can tilt your pelvis in a detrimental way for your curve type. Ask your Schroth therapist for postural guidance.

Set up your workspace

- Use a standing adjustable desk if possible.
- DOCUMENT HOLDER/BOOK: Next to and at the same height as the monitor.
- SCREEN: 0-20º below the horizon of sight, slightly below eye level. Place your monitor 18-22" away from your body (about arm's length). Screen should be free of glare and should pivot, blue light filter if possible.
- KEYBOARD: Same height as elbows with wrists slightly bent.
- MOUSE: Next to and at the same height as the keyboard.
- HEAD/NECK/EYES: the head is back, chin tucked and ears/shoulders/hips aligned. 20-28º viewing angle (Level with the top of the screen)
- ELBOWS: 90-100º angle at sides
- ARMS: Minimal bend at the wrist, sometimes no armrest is best, as it lets arms fall naturally.
- LOWER BACK: Support lumbar curve
- HIPS: 90-120º angle
- SITTING BONES: Equal pressure
- FEET: Flat on the floor or on a footrest
- CHAIR: Supports your back from the pelvis to the shoulder blades. Adjustable so your feet are flat on the floor and your knees are bent slightly more than 90˚ in front of you.
- Try a theraball for sitting which is helpful for balance and muscle activation.
- Take breaks every 30 minutes.

Your Schroth practitioner may have made specific recommendations on how you should sit for your specific curve situation. Follow it as closely as you can.

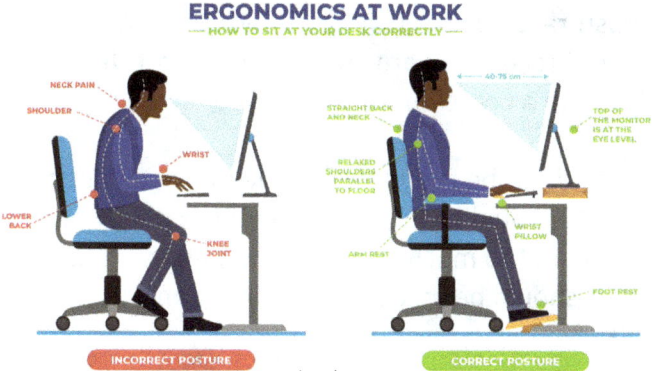

ERGONOMICS AT WORK
— HOW TO SIT AT YOUR DESK CORRECTLY —

NECK PAIN

SHOULDER

WRIST

LOWER BACK

KNEE JOINT

INCORRECT POSTURE

40-75 cm

STRAIGHT BACK AND NECK

TOP OF THE MONITOR IS AT THE EYE LEVEL

RELAXED SHOULDERS PARALLEL TO FLOOR

WRIST PILLOW

ARM REST

FOOT REST

CORRECT POSTURE

Image by Freepik

12. EXERCISE AND SCOLIOSIS (SCHROTH)

If you wear a brace you will remove it to perform any scoliosis-specific postural exercises (SSPE) or physical therapy. You will also remove your brace if you are involved in a sport that would be impossible with a brace on.

Bracing should not be used alone in the management of idiopathic scoliosis. SSPE should be incorporated. If the prescribed exercise protocols create too much stress for the patient, then adjustments should be made in the bracing and/or the exercise schedule.

As explained in Chapter 11 "What Should I Avoid," high-impact activities are not recommended.

Things to focus on
- Strength is vital to improving or halting curve progression and reducing pain. Exercise, even non-specific scoliosis-based exercise, is beneficial for scoliosis and can have a positive effect.
- Elongation of the spine with postural correction and actual traction unless there is a fusion. Traction stretch helps with pain and general discomfort.
- Working and lengthening of muscles in the concavities of the spine.
- Restoration of the sagittal curves (front to back). Avoid extension or flexion where the curves are already reduced or magnified.

- Avoid rotation or side bending as the spine already likely has side bend and rotational issues.

- Breathing into the concavities (inside of the curve) causes the ribs to work as levers to de-rotate the spine AND improve pulmonary function.

- Core work

- Balance/sense of body position.

- Stretching muscles: hamstrings, quadriceps and hip flexor muscles can increase hip flexibility and can be a substitute for a loss in spine mobility and make it easier to move in desired directions.

- Encourage spinal articulation: open the spinal joints in the fixated areas to reduce stiffness.

- Activities of daily living to improve posture all the time, not just during exercises.

- Play low-impact sports.

- Choose exercises carefully based on curves and consult with a skilled scoliosis practitioner.

Scoliosis Specific Postural Exercise (SSPE)
Scoliosis-specific postural exercises such as Schroth, etc., outlined in Chapter 6 "Alternative Treatments," improve the strength of the trunk, reduce asymmetric spinal loading and improve postural awareness. These exercises also address the front-to-back (sagittal curves) of the spine to create a healthy "spring" for the spine and take the stress off of scoliosis. A very important part of any program is knowing what habits and exercises or sports may

affect the sagittal curves. This will help you make the best choices and modifications in your daily life.

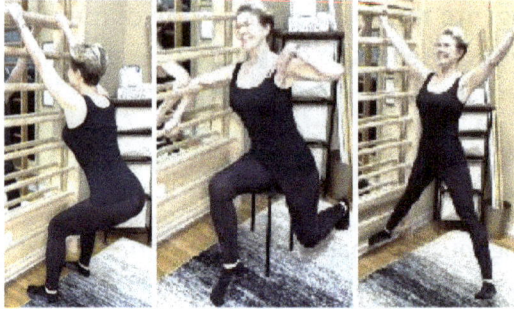

Scoliosis Specific (Schroth) Exercises

Text Neck/Forward Head Carriage/Scoli Neck Exercises

- The goal is to align the head over the neck
- Use proper ergonomics (work/school/cell phone)
- Perform Z Translation exercises
- Perform chest stretches
- Curve restoration with a neck fulcrum device or a small 3-4" foam roller.
- Proper pillow for sleeping to support the neck curvature

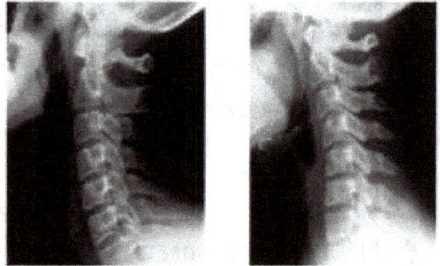

Normal Neck alignment / Flattened Neck Alignment

Fulcrum Work

A cervical neck fulcrum device is easy to use for 3-10 minutes a day and is highly recommended by chiropractors for neck, shoulder and upper back pain and forward head carriage. Rest over the device for stretching, alignment correcting and neck curve restoration.

154

3 options:
1. Core Products Apex Cervical Orthosis. Has graduated levels as the foam breaks apart to create less or more intensity.
2. Restorative Cervical Traction Neck Fulcrum Wedge Pillow. This device has various positions to create less or more intensity.
3. White Round Foam Roller, 4" X 12" (adult) 3" X 12" (child). A cost-effective, simple and space-saving way to create not only curve creation but slight traction due to the ability to "spin" the roller into position.

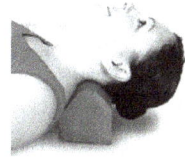

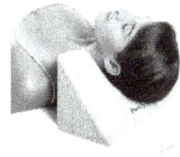

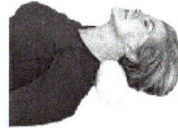

Fulcrum rehab exercises are necessary to complete and maintain spine and posture correction.

Fulcrum Exercises

Lie supine with the neck device in place, (option to use a lumbar curve pillow). The neck will now be in extension. Hold the extension for the following movements.

- Place hands on thighs to create pressure against legs while the neck is in extension.

- Then the neck is in extension with rotation on both sides.

- Then the neck is in extension with a neck side bend on both sides.

Press with hands against legs and hold each position for 5 seconds.
10 times in each position.
Add wedging and directional breathing if prescribed by a Schroth therapist.

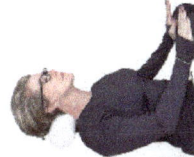

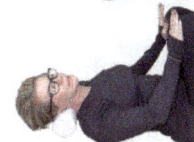

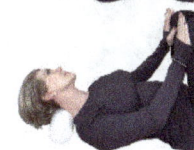

Z Translation Movement ("chicken")

Seated upright in neutral alignment (head over shoulders, etc.). Retracting the chin from neutral alignment: pull the chin back to the base of the skull.

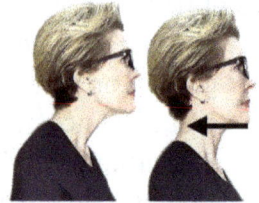

"Chicken with a Ball": While seated, place a soft 5-8" ball directly behind the head against a wall to perform "retractions" of pulling the chin to the base of the skull (don't tilt the chin down or tilt the head back). Press slowly and hold for 1-3 counts and slowly release to neutral (not forward). Repeat 10 times, rest and repeat 3 sets. Stop with any pain.

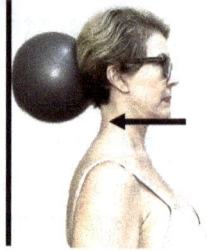

Cervical Stretches

These should be performed slowly and carefully to the point where a stretch is felt but with no pain. There should be no bouncing. If the stretches increase pain or create any symptoms, stop. Sit up straight, sit on your hands with palms up, or the hands can hold under the chair for additional stretch. Lift thru the crown of the head. Never jam the neck. Perform a slight tuck of chin/retraction ("chicken") to begin.

1.   Rotation: Gently turn the head left to hold and breathe 5-10 seconds. Repeat on the right, aiming to align the chin over the shoulder.

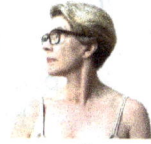

2.   Flexion / Extension: a nod to chest then chin lifts to ceiling. Back to neutral.

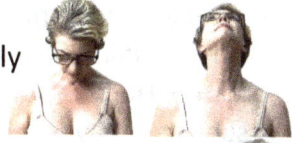

3.   Lateral: Head in neutral posture, gently bring ear to shoulder and hold for 5-10 seconds. Repeat on the opposite side, gently, never to the point of pain. Back to neutral.

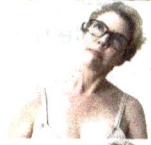

4.   Diagonal Posterior Neck: Head tilted down, gently bring ear to shoulder slowly and breathe and hold for 5-10 seconds. Repeat on the opposite side. Back to neutral.

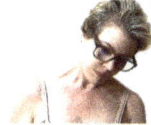

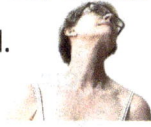

5.   Diagonal Anterior Neck: Head tilted back, gently bring ear to shoulder. Breathe and hold for 5-10 seconds. Repeat on the opposite side. Back to neutral.

6.   Levator Scapulae Stretch: Seated tall neutral spine and neck, place a hand gently on top of the head elbow pointed at the same knee, rotate the head to line up the chin with the knee, with the weight of the hand only, gently stretch towards the knee then slowly rotate chin inward and then outward. Breathe and hold for 5-10 seconds. Release gently.

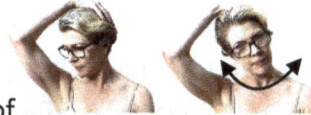

Note: Do stretches slowly, always rise thru the crown of the head and never to the point of pain.

Cervical Isometric Strengthening Exercises

Begin by sitting up with the head in the best possible alignment stacked over the shoulders and" chicken" the chin over the chest. Lengthen the entire spine and neck. The key to isometric exercise is to strengthen the muscles without moving. Resist the pressure while maintaining constant tension in the neck muscles. Be sure to breathe. Holding your breath may cause an increase in blood pressure that may result in your becoming dizzy or lightheaded.

1.   Side neck muscles: Head held neutral. Place your palm against the right side of your head (temple area). Take a deep breath through the nose and press against the side of the head for 5 seconds. Have your head match the resistance on the right side without bringing your ear towards the shoulder. Switch sides.

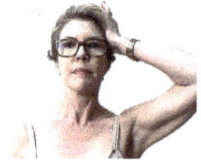

2.   Front neck muscles: Head held neutral. Place the palms of your hands on the front of your forehead. Take a deep breath through the nose and isometrically press on the forehead for 5 seconds. Have your forehead match the resistance of your palms. Breathe out slowly through your mouth.
Variation: Placed laced hands under the chin and press up lifting and lengthening the neck.

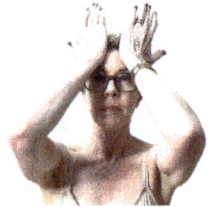

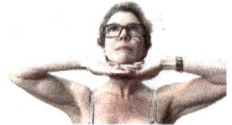

3.   Back neck muscles: Head held neutral. Clasp your hands behind the back of your head. Take a deep breath through the nose to press the back of your head against your hands for 5 seconds. Have your head match the resistance of your palms. Breathe out slowly through your mouth.

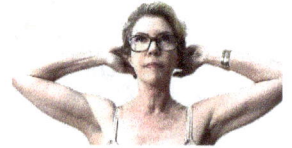

4. Rotational neck muscles: Turn your head to the side. Place a hand on the jaw across the cheek. Take a deep breath through the nose to press the face rotationally against your hand for 5 seconds. Have your head match the resistance of your palm. Breathe out slowly through your mouth.
Chin lift - repeat as above but add a slight chin lift repeat the slight pressure and isometric hold.
Chin tuck - repeat as above but add a slight chin down repeat the slight pressure and isometric hold. Reverse and repeat all on the opposite side.

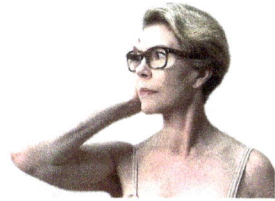

Compression Techniques
Foam Roll/Tennis or Therapy Balls. Press the roll or ball against any particular sore spot and BREATHE until tenderness decreases by 70%. (20-30 seconds). Not to be done with fusions, surgery, or disease of the area. Trigger points are knotty, involuntary contractions of muscle bundles. They prevent the muscle from relaxing and recovering.

Neck

High Neck Tennis Ball Massage:

2 tennis/therapy balls taped together or in a sock, etc.:

Lying on your back with knees bent, place a yoga block under the head, place balls on top of the block at the base of the skull:

- Feel neck traction, relax and move the balls to the sore spot as needed.

- Then perform a chin up and down "yes" action.

- Then turn the head side to side in a" no" action.

- You may hold anywhere during the "no" and add the "yes" motion to work any sore areas.

- Then back to neutral again to now rotate the nose in an "Infinity" pattern, or a "Figure 8" in a side-to-side direction and reverse.

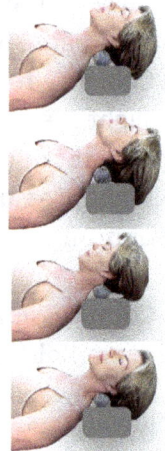

Low Neck Tennis Balls:

2 separate tennis balls across the top of the upper back muscles:

Lying on your back with knees bent, place a yoga block under the head and then the two balls behind your upper back muscles:

- Arms wave up and around in "wave-like movements" toward the ceiling.

- Reach arms straight to the ceiling, palms facing in. On an inhale reach and then exhale to pull back the shoulders.

- Bear Hug: Cross your arms over your body giving yourself a bear hug and "wiggle" the upper body to massage the area.

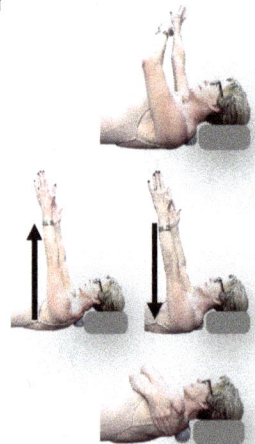

Upper Back

We will assume there is a flattened upper back curve (loss of kyphosis) and a flattened low back curve (loss of lordosis) for these techniques unless noted.

Foam Roller Release Routine

To release the spine and ribs which hold the scoliotic pattern in place. Ideally, perform these exercises before and after any physical activity. Avoid rolling over the kidney area.

1. For a flat or lordotic thoracic spine, the goal is to maintain spinal flexion and stay slightly rounded in the spine. *Do NOT perform a backbend over the roller.* While supine on the horizontal roller, support the head in hands, hips up and abs engaged. Roll up and down the spine but no lower than the lowest ribs. Perform again on either side of the spinal musculature by slightly rotating off-center (right or left). The areas on the convex side will usually be sorer and tighter.

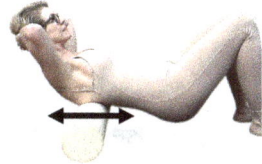

2. For a kyphotic thoracic spine, the goal is to allow a slight extension of the upper spine.

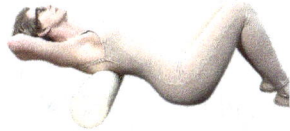

3. Roll the serratus, latissimus and teres muscles by lying laterally on the roller under the armpit (support the head with your hands) and roll up/down in a small range of motion from the tricep to just below the armpit. Find any sore area and hold to roll slightly front/back on the area.

This will be most useful under the armpit of the convex side of the spine to release the tight muscles holding the shoulder girdle.

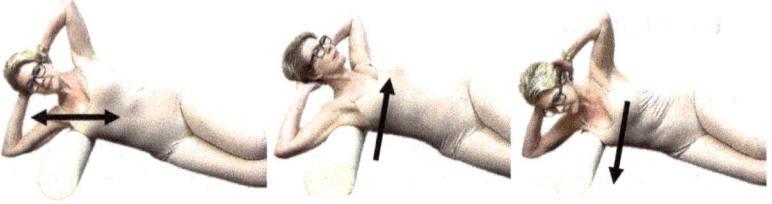

Traction Work
Apply the breath work here and use caution with shoulder issues. To provide an elongation of the spine: to stretch spinal muscles in preparation for exercise; to obtain pain relief and to open discs; and to find sagittal curves in a relaxed position.

You can use anything secure such as:
Doorway, sink, ballet barre, chin-up bar, heavy gym equipment. Get creative and always brace the equipment.

1. Flat Upper Thoracic Spine - hands grasp solid objects at shoulder height or higher. Bend the knees to pull away into the "chair" position, elongate the spine and pull the hips back. The head should not fall between the arms.
If you have a flat upper back then you want to round it. If you have a flat lower back then you want to arch it. Breath - Inhale into the flattened concave areas to open them. Do not allow flattened thoracic or lumbar areas to become more so.

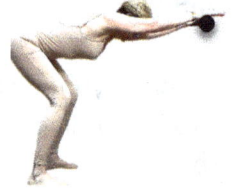

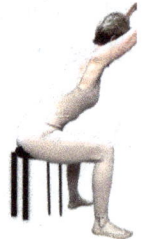

Modification: sit down in a chair and reach as high up as possible to create the stretch.

162

2. Kyphotic Upper Thoracic Spine - hands grasp a solid object at shoulder height or higher. Bend the knees to pull away into the "chair" position, elongate the spine and pull the hips back. Head lifts and chest may fall between the arms toward the floor. Breath - Inhale into the sides and front of the body. We want sagittal curves to be improved as needed. Chest/ribs forward and lower back arched or tucked pelvis as needed.

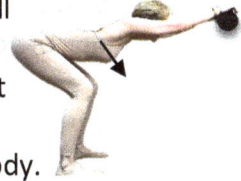

McKenzie/Extension Type Exercises

Extension is good for the lumbar spine since we want to encourage lordosis when the low back arch is reduced. Take caution with the range of motion. Work within neutral and venture carefully into flexion or extension and monitor the reaction the next day or so.

Example: Cobra exercise, performed when there is a flat upper thoracic spine, should be modified in the following way:

1. Face down with elbows bent, palms down just under the chest and retract shoulders.
2. Arch the upper spine into a "dolphin shape" and extend the spine with a focus into the lower back as a "mini cobra" is performed to create a rounding of the upper back. Breathe into flattened/concave areas of the spine. Lower and repeat. Option: shift the ribs away from the "bump" of the scoliosis in the thoracic spine.

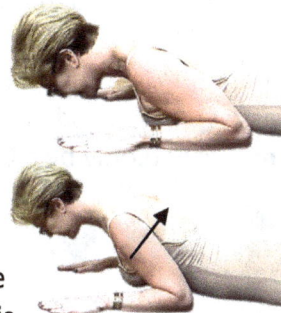

Cobra for a kyphotic upper thoracic spine:
1. Face down with elbows bent, palms down just under the chest, retract shoulders
2. Perform a traditional cobra with extension in the upper back. The chest will lift forward. Breathe into the front of the ribs. Option: shift the ribs away from the "bump" of the scoliosis of the thoracic spine.

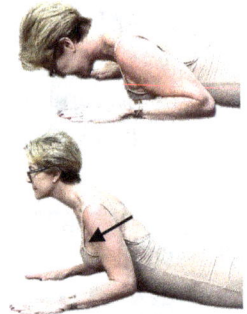

Padding Discussion
Scoliosis can cause your legs to appear to be different lengths making you want to pad under a leg, foot, hip, etc. Trying to level a leg or hip can cause more harm than good. A full explanation of the hidden curves and rotations that occur in the pelvis needs to be made by a professional therapist. You should never attempt to pad a pelvis or "short leg" without a therapist's guidance. Padding will affect ALL of the curves sagittal and frontal and is COMPLEX. Your scoliosis practitioner/therapist may give you specific wedges or pillows to use with your specific scoliosis. This is different for each person so there is no value in following a generic guide that was not prescribed for you. Be sure to follow your wedge instructions carefully. Add them to your daily life such as your workouts, resting, or sleeping. Wedging properly can reduce pain, assist a brace and give postural support. Wedges should be prescribed only by a trained scoliosis professional.

Breathing With Scoliosis

With scoliosis, the spine bends and rotates. One side becomes shortened and compressed, while the other becomes extended and strained outward. Imagine the lungs and heart inside a compressed left rib area.

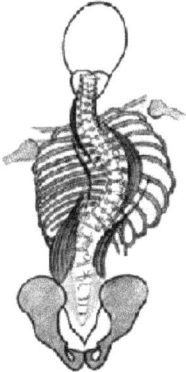

Convexity (outer edge of curve)
Causes over-extended muscles with decreased muscle contractive capacity and expanded ribs. These muscles are tight.

Concavity (inner edge of curve)
Causes short atrophied muscles and closed ribs, airspace and lungs. These muscles are weak.

THIS IS AN EXAMPLE OF A RIGHT THORACIC CURVE AND A LEFT LUMBAR CURVE. IT MAY BE REVERSED IN SOME CASES

With scoliosis, there is often a decreased breathing capacity on the inside of the curve (concave side) because the ribs may be compressed together and the muscles along the spine and between the ribs lose some of their elasticity and strength.

Breathing into the compressed ribcage on the concave side creates more lung capacity and oxygenates the body, lengthens the spine, de-rotates the ribcage, strengthens the muscles on this weaker side, creates more evenness of the sides of the body and relieves pain. This directional asymmetrical breath can correct or prevent further progression of the curvature and is a critical part of a therapeutic program. Even if it is as simple as adding a deep breath during the workday or commute, breathing into the concave areas is very impactful.

If correct breathing is neglected, the breathing may automatically default into the convex/larger area and the curve can get worse. Always work with an experienced therapist and know how to modify your practice for your scoliosis.

Scoliosis Breathing Lab

Focus the inhale to stretch the concave or flat areas where the ribs are closed. This can be learned by lying down face up, seated, or standing. Use a band wrapped around the area to provide tactile feedback.

If lying face up, use any prescribed scoliosis wedging and proceed. Breathe into these compressed/collapsed areas of the ribs as if to "Smell a Flower" or "Inflate like a Balloon" or touch the area to feel the inflation. Repeat this technique during your daily routine, during exercise, or during scoliosis-specific postural exercises to reap huge benefits.

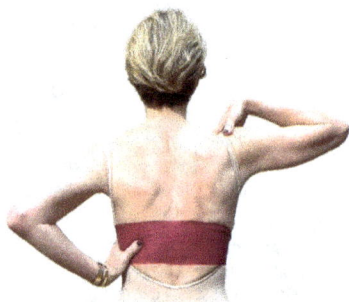

Kyphosis Breathing Lab

Just like in scoliosis, a hyperkyphotic spine needs length and strength and the spine needs the ribs to open in the compressed areas. The front becomes shortened and compressed, while the upper back becomes extended and strained outward. This breathing can be practiced while lying face up, seated, or standing. Use a band wrapped around the area to provide tactile feedback. If lying face up, use any prescribed scoliosis wedging and proceed. Take a deep breath ("smell a flower") into the front and side ribs (forward, out and up). Think:" Pushing your lowest front ribs forward," lift the chin slightly and slightly tuck the pelvis under.

13. NUTRITION AND SUPPLEMENTS

Always consult with your doctor before starting any supplementation or diet.

A contribution from Erin O'Bryan, Holistic Health Coach
hello@erinobryanchc.com. http://erinobryanchc.com

We have all heard that food is medicine and that food can help heal us. So how does this apply to scoliosis? I examine this in detail below. However, to start, go get yourself tested. If you have scoliosis, there's a good chance that you have a hormonal or nutritional imbalance. In this chapter, I address a variety of nutritional and hormonal imbalances that can have an impact on scoliosis. The good news? How you can correct them. Correcting these imbalances can have a positive effect on overall well-being and spinal health. If your physician is not able to order these tests, consult with a naturopath or functional medicine doctor. There are several important nutritional and herbal supplements that support bone health. Supporting bone health is especially important for those with scoliosis as bone loss conditions such as osteoporosis, osteopenia and low bone density, have been proven to lead to scoliosis progression. Below are a variety of vitamins and minerals that are essential to bone health:

Vitamin D
You can support your bone health by testing your vitamin D levels (a simple blood test your doctor can order). If your levels are low, your doctor will prescribe the appropriate supplementation. Supplementation with vitamin D usually comes in the form of D3, as studies have repeatedly shown that vitamin D3 is superior at raising levels of vitamin D in the body.

Why Vitamin D? Vitamin D helps your body absorb calcium and phosphorus, both of which are essential for bone health. Vitamin D also modulates your body's inflammatory response. As a result, when your levels are low, your osteoclasts (cells that remove old bone) begin to work at an accelerated rate. This means you start losing old bone faster than your osteoblasts (cells that build new bone) can replace it. Studies show that higher levels of vitamin D stimulate your osteoblasts which is why low levels of vitamin D are associated with osteomalacia, osteopenia and osteoporosis.

The National Institutes of Health recommends that adults get 600 to 800 IUs of vitamin D daily, children 600 IUs and infants 400IUs. The amount of IUs in your supplement will depend upon your levels as shown by your blood test. Your doctor or other qualified healthcare professional can advise you. Vitamin D is a fat-soluble vitamin, which means it is absorbed in the bloodstream best in the presence of dietary fat. Take your vitamin D with a meal that contains healthy fat for the best absorption.

You can also get vitamin D from your food choices. Foods that contain the highest levels of vitamin D include fatty fish such as wild-caught salmon, trout, shrimp, tuna, sardines and fish oils, such as cod liver oil. Cereals and milk are often fortified with vitamin D. Even mushrooms and egg yolks contain some vitamin D. As an example, if you have a 3.5-ounce serving of salmon at dinner you will be receiving roughly 350 IUs of vitamin D. Sun exposure is also the body's way of making its own vitamin D. Proponents who have studied this method have found that 10 to 15 minutes of sun exposure to a mostly bare body, at noon, twice a week, will provide all the vitamin D a person needs. However, current recommendations of the American Academy of Dermatology argue against this method of obtaining vitamin D citing that the risk of skin cancer from such exposure outweighs the benefit, particularly since vitamin D can be found in food and supplement form. So why risk it?

Calcium

We all know that calcium is important to bone health, but how to put it to work in your bones has changed over the years. As you read above, vitamin D is crucial to this task. If you don't have enough vitamin D your body won't utilize whatever calcium may be in your system.

The calcium requirement for children 1-3 years is 700 mg, 4-8-year-olds need 1,000 mg and 9-18-year-olds require 1,300 mg. For adult men, the requirement is 1,000 mg and after age 70, it goes up to 1,200 mg. For women, the recommended dosage goes from 1,000 mg to 1,200 after age 50. Food sources of calcium are abundant as you will see with a quick internet search. A few of the big ones are dairy products, leafy greens and canned fish. And don't worry, if you avoid dairy, most dairy substitutes are fortified with calcium, making it easy to boost your daily calcium intake. Calcium supplements are also better absorbed when taken in small doses (500 mg or less) at different times during the day. And in most people, calcium supplements are better absorbed when taken with food.

Vitamin K2

Vitamin K, like vitamin D, also helps you absorb calcium effectively. Specifically, it activates a protein – osteocalcin – that helps calcium get into your bones and it also activates something called the matrix GLA protein, which prevents calcium from building up in soft tissues. Without vitamin K, calcium may not get to the right place and may even cause problems by accumulating somewhere it's not supposed to be, like the kidneys or blood vessels.

Vitamin K exists in two forms: K1 and K2. K2 is the one thought to be most effective for supplementation.

Good food sources of K2 are fermented foods like nattō (whole, fermented soybeans) and sauerkraut and some animal sources like liver, egg yolks and chicken. Our gut bacteria also produce some vitamin K2, when we have a healthy microbiome (gut environment). Some dietary K1 is also converted to K2 in the gut as well. Like vitamin D, vitamin K is fat-soluble meaning its best absorbed when taken along with some form of fat. The Adequate Intake (AI) of vitamin K2 for adult men is 120 mcg daily and 90 mcg for women. More research is needed on vitamin K. For now, the AI is the minimal amount needed to prevent a deficiency.

Magnesium

Simply put, magnesium converts vitamin D into its active form so it can aid calcium absorption. Magnesium has a whole host of other very important roles in good health and, sadly, about one-half of all Americans are deficient in this important mineral. The RDA for magnesium is about 300 mg a day, however, most people benefit from 400 to 1,000 mg a day. The most absorbable forms are magnesium citrate, glycinate, taurate, or aspartate. Avoid magnesium carbonate, sulfate, gluconate and oxide because they are not well absorbed in the body.

Side effects from too much magnesium include diarrhea which can often be avoided if you switch to magnesium glycinate. People with kidney disease or severe heart disease should take magnesium only under a doctor's supervision.

Strontium

Strontium is a mineral primarily found in seawater and soil. You get it mainly from seafood and in lesser amounts in whole milk, wheat bran, beef, poultry and root vegetables. Strontium is found in supplement form such as strontium citrate or strontium ranelate. I advise avoiding strontium ranelate which has been shown to have numerous harmful side effects including heart attacks and blood clots. Strontium citrate, as opposed to strontium ranelate, is a safe form of strontium and has been shown to positively influence the biomarkers associated with slowing osteopenia. And this can be a better solution for males as compared with calcium supplementation which increases the risks of prostate calcification.

Strontium Citrate
It has been discovered that strontium citrate may have a greater affinity for bone matrix than calcium. Thus, there may be a benefit to adding it to the regime of vitamin D and vitamin K2. Strontium is similar to calcium. It seems to play a role in how your body makes new bone while it slows the breakdown of old bone, which means it may affect how strong your bones are. Some research shows that women with osteoporosis may not absorb strontium as they should which could be a contributing factor the osteoporosis.

Grape Seed Extract
Grape seed extract (not to be confused with grapefruit seed extract) is a dietary supplement made by removing, drying and pulverizing the seeds of grapes. Grape seeds are rich in antioxidants, including flavonoids. Antioxidants are beneficial to the body in numerous ways. In terms of bone health, a few promising animal studies have shown that increasing flavonoid consumption may improve collagen synthesis and bone formation. As a rich source of flavonoids, grape seed extract may thus help increase your bone density and strength. Animal studies have found that adding grape seed extract to either a low, standard, or high calcium diet can increase bond density, mineral content and bone strength. More research needs to be done

before dosage recommendations can be made for specific health purposes. However, doses ranging from 100 to 400 mg have been used in most studies. Talk with your doctor first if you are considering using grape seed extract.

The Role of Inflammation in Scoliosis
Controlling inflammation in the body can also have a huge impact on the development and progression of scoliosis. Here's how this works: The immune system becomes activated when the body recognizes anything foreign, whether it's an invading microbe, plant pollen, or chemical. This in turn triggers a process called inflammation. And intermittent inflammation directed at these truly threatening invaders protects the body. When inflammation persists daily, even when no foreign invader is threatening, then inflammation becomes harmful.

It has been found that inflammation in the body may lead to scoliosis progression and degeneration at any age. Research is also pointing towards the immune response as the mechanism responsible for tissue changes associated with scoliosis curvature progression.

Inflammation can be regulated through nutritional changes by adding supplements and eliminating foods that cause inflammation.

So, what are these **bad foods** that cause inflammation?

- Processed foods, which include most fast food, like French fries, onion rings, burgers, etc.
- Sugar is one of the biggest offenders here. Not just candy and desserts. Sugar sneaks into all kinds of foods like bread, salad dressing and sauces, so be sure to read food labels.
- Alcohol

172

- Margarine, shortening, lard (unhealthy fats)
- Processed meat such as hot dogs, sausage and bacon
- Refined carbohydrates such as white bread, white rice and bagels (Always opt for 100% whole grain)
- Soda and other sugar-sweetened beverages (Again – sugar!).

Be proactive and load your diet with anti-inflammatory foods. Basically, this includes whole foods, healthy fats and especially whole grains. The Mediterranean Diet is an excellent whole food, anti-inflammatory way of eating. Many websites and cookbooks make it easy to follow the Mediterranean Diet.

Fruits and vegetables such as blueberries, apples and leafy greens that are high in natural antioxidants and polyphenols (protective compounds found in plants) are excellent anti-inflammatory foods to consume daily.

Here are some other great **anti-inflammatory food** choices:
- Tomatoes
- Olive oil
- Avocado oil
- Spinach, kale and collards
- Nuts
- Fatty fish like salmon, mackerel, tuna and sardines
- Coffee and tea

Botanical supplements have also been clinically shown to reduce inflammation and can be found in supplement form:
- Curcumin, which is found in turmeric. Research supports that combining the piperine in black pepper with the curcumin

in turmeric enhances curcumin absorption by up to 2,000%, so make sure your turmeric supplement has piperine.

- Saffron
- Quercetin dihydrate is a plant flavonoid polyphenol that also shows strong effects on immunity and inflammation. It is found in many fruits, vegetables, seeds and grains. A few of the common foods highest in quercetin are capers, red onions and kale. It can also be taken as a supplement.
- Grape Seed Extract (as mentioned above) has been shown to improve bone health in animal studies and is a powerful antioxidant as well.
- Fish oil supplements are also an excellent source for their anti-inflammatory properties.

Hormones
The role of hormones in the development and progression of scoliosis is still being actively studied. Here is some of what we now know….

Melatonin
Some new studies are showing a connection between sleep, melatonin and bone health. Melatonin is a hormone that is released during sleep and promotes a healthy sleep-wake cycle. It is during sleep that the brain also releases human growth hormone. So if not enough melatonin is secreted, sleep is not of great quality and consequently, not enough growth hormone is secreted and proper growth is not supported.

Recent research in mice has shown that melatonin deficiency plays a crucial role in the development of scoliosis. The research has also shown that the restoration of melatonin levels helps to enhance low bond density, correct abnormal bone quality and arrest the development and progression of the scoliotic deformity

174

in mice. Recent research has also found that postmenopausal women who got less than 5 hours of sleep a night have lower bone mineral density than those who sleep 7 or more hours. Researchers believe the lack of sleep interferes with bone remodeling that happens when you sleep.

Melatonin levels can be measured with a blood test. Supplementation should only be considered under a doctor's supervision, especially for children. To encourage melatonin production and a good night's sleep, a regular sleep routine should be established and the bedroom should be as dark as possible, particularly free from blue light (cell phones and computers). Sleep routines include no blue light devices up to an hour or two before bedtime, going to bed at the same time each night, sleeping in a cool room, engaging in a relaxing, soothing activity 30 minutes to one hour before bedtime such as reading and again, a room as dark as possible.

Progesterone
A few recent studies, including one in 2022, suggest a potential relationship between low levels of progesterone and idiopathic scoliosis among females. Progesterone levels can be revealed via a blood test and, again, supplementation with progesterone should only be done in consultation with a physician.

Estrogen
The exact role of estrogen in adolescent idiopathic scoliosis (AIS) and its mechanisms are controversial. Further research is needed to determine the exact roles and mechanisms by which estrogen participates in the onset and progression of adolescent idiopathic scoliosis.

Menopause and Scoliosis

There are two ways in which women in menopause can suffer from degenerative scoliosis. The first is a progression of previously diagnosed scoliosis during menopause. The second instance is where scoliosis develops during peri-menopause or menopause. More studies need to be done on the topic but degenerative scoliosis is likely the result of the decline in hormones, particularly estrogen, during this stage of life.

What is well documented is that the significant declines in estrogen experienced during the menopause transition contribute to accelerated bone loss. Hormone therapy reverses bone loss and helps prevent fractures. During the first three years of hormone therapy use, bone density has been shown to increase steadily and then is maintained during continued use. Consultation with your doctor is important before beginning hormone therapy.

Women who are approaching menopause or post-menopausal can help prevent degenerative scoliosis by using weights and performing load-bearing exercises, both of which are proven to increase bone density. It is also especially important at this stage to take the supplements recommended above consistently and follow a healthy, anti-inflammatory diet.

Summary

The combination of consistent supplementation, an anti-inflammatory diet and regular exercise, are all some of your best bets for easing your symptoms and staving off the progression of scoliosis.

14. CHOOSING A DOCTOR

Choosing an Orthopedist or Spine Specialist/Neurologist
You probably learned about scoliosis through a routine exam or observed a posture imbalance and went to the doctor to check it out. The likely first step is imaging such as an X-ray. A measurement of the curves and skeletal age is done first.
From here you will begin to make choices of what route you go and with what doctor. Once you have been sent to the orthopedist or spine specialist this will likely be your point person to guide you through the entire journey. Choose this doctor carefully. A second or third opinion is a terrific idea. Choosing a doctor that you are comfortable with is vital since I and many of my colleagues have heard unfortunate stories of some medical doctors being less than supportive of their concerned and vulnerable patients. Also, dismissing and not addressing a curvature is risky as a curve can rapidly progress in younger people. This is the "watch and what" approach that was discussed in Chapter 9 "Bracing". Be proactive and find a like-minded doctor. The following are some topics to consider when choosing or working with a doctor.

Find a doctor who is:

- Board Certified
- Who specializes in the treatment of pediatric and teenage spinal deformities.
- Is affiliated with a hospital.
- Has a staff experienced in caring for patients during and after spinal surgery?
- Has successful experience treating pediatric or adult spinal deformities.
- Has references

If a child is younger than 10 and the curve is 10º or larger, a referral to an orthopedist or a spine specialist is necessary.

If a child is older than 10 years and the curve is 20º or larger, is combined with any back pain or neurological issues, a referral to an orthopedist, spine specialist, or neurologist is necessary.

Visual Assessment
The doctor should perform a visual assessment along with the imaging.

- Measure the patient's height.
- Check the shoulders and hips for asymmetry.
- Check for leg length discrepancies.
- Patients who are tall with long fingers and an increased arm span-to-height ratio should be assessed for other signs of Marfan syndrome (Such as cardiac abnormalities).
- Patients with joint and skin hyper-laxity along with scoliosis may need to have further workup for a connective tissue condition such as Ehlers-Danlos syndrome.
- High-arched or cavus feet may be associated with a neurological disorder such as Charcot-Marie-Tooth disease or a spinal cord abnormality such as a tumor.
- Skin inspection that notes café-au-lait spots or armpit freckles suggests neurofibromatosis.
- A hairy patch or skin dimpling in the back may identify a myelomeningocele (the most serious type of spina bifida. With this condition, a sac of fluid comes through an opening in the baby's back. Part of the spinal cord and nerves are in this sac and are damaged).

Gauging the pubertal development is done with imaging but also with Tanner Staging which is a visual assessment of a child. See Tables 1 and 2.

Table 1	Tanner Staging Females			
Tanner Stage	Breasts	Pubic Hair	Growth	Other
1	Elevation of papilla only	Villus hair only	2-2.4 inches per year	Adrenarche and ovarian growth
2	Breast bud under areola, areola enlargement	Sparse hair along the labia	2.8-3.2 inches per year	Clitoral enlargement, labia pigmentation, growth of uterus
3	Breast tissue grows but has no contour or separation	Course hair curled pigmented covers the pubes	3.2 inches per year	Axillary hair, acne
4	Projection of areola and papilla, secondary mound formation	Adult hair, does not spread to the thigh	2.8 inches per year	Menarche and development of menses
5	Adult type contour, projection of papilla only	Adult hair, spreads to the medial thigh	Cessation of linear growth	Adult genitalia

Table 2	Tanner Staging Males			
Tanner Stage	Genitalia	Pubic Hair	Growth	Other
1	Testes <2.5 cm	Villus hair only	2.0-2.4 inches per year	Adrenarche
2	Testes 2.5.-3.2 cm Thinning and reddening of the scrotum	Sparse hair at penis base	2.0-2.4 inches per year	Decrease in body fat
3	Testes 3.3-4.0 cm Increase of penis length	Thicker curly hair spreads to the pubis	2.8-3.2 inches per year	Gynecomastia, voice break, increased muscle mass
4	Testes 4.1-4.5 cm Penis Measure , darkening of scrotum	Adult hair does not spread to thighs	4.0 inches per year	Axillary hair, voice change, acne
5	Testes >4.5 cm Adult genitalia	Adult hair spreads to medial thigh	Deceleration, cessation	Facial hair, muscle mass increase

Neurological Exam
Since some scoliosis cases can be caused by neuromuscular conditions as described in previous chapters, your doctor must perform a complete neurological examination to evaluate balance, reflexes and motor testing and sensory testing of the lower extremities, back and chest. This is especially important if

scoliosis is visualized on imaging but has no measurable rotation using a scoliometer on the Adam's forward bending test. Side note: The inability to perform this test due to pain in the back or hamstring tightness can suggest other pathology, including mechanical back pain, disc herniation, spondylolysis, or infection.

Other Imaging May Be Needed
An MRI study may be ordered by the doctor as a follow-up to the X-ray to make sure scoliosis does not have any underlying causes that need to be ruled out. This is the standard of care if the person is under 10 years old and also if the curve is to the left in the upper (Thoracic) spine.

A Note on The Forward Bending/Adams Test by Schools and Doctors:

Some states in the US require schools to screen children for Scoliosis using the forward bending test. This is usually done in adolescents between 5-7th grades. It may be performed by the school nurse, a coach, the physical education teacher, or a physician may be brought into the school.

The Scoliosis Research Society (USA) recommends annual screening of all children between 10 and 14 years of age. The American Academy of Pediatrics recommends screening at routine health visits at 10, 12, 14 and 16 years of age.

The US Preventive Services Task Force and the Canadian Task Force concluded that there was insufficient evidence to recommend for or against the screening of adolescents. Most jurisdictions have unfortunately abandoned routine screening and many cases of scoliosis have gone undiagnosed.

Dos & Don'ts

Dos:

- Be prepared to be overwhelmed with new information and documentation to keep track of.

- Start a notebook to keep all of your information in one place and also to make notes.

- Get information about your curvature and learn about all the options available to you and don't stop at the first bit of information you receive.

- Work out a way forward and find the strategies and techniques that best suit you and resonate with your gut feeling.

- Look at all of your options and make informed decisions.

Don'ts:

- Do not be afraid to ask questions

- Do not allow yourself to be pushed into a treatment or surgery that you are not ready for or are not comfortable with.

We need to gain knowledge and understanding of our scoliosis to learn the tools and explore our options. Knowledge is power. Many people seeking medical care just accept what the doctor suggests and they don't explore other options in a very important decision.

Choosing a physical therapist or scoliosis-specific postural exercise practitioner

If you choose to go the route of exercise therapy, choosing this person will be as important of a decision as it was with any other physician. Questions and topics to help choose your Schroth or scoliosis-specific postural exercise therapist may include:

- Asking how long the practitioner has been using the method and if they are full or part-time using the method.

- What method do they use and have you researched this method?

- Will your insurance cover it or is this an out-of-pocket cost?

- Was this person referred by your physician or by a personal referral or internet search? Have you read reviews?

- Is the therapist going to be working with you or are you going to be with an aide or in a large class setting? You may want more specialized attention.

- Do they require you to use chiropractic adjustments as part of the therapy? Many do not wish to add this as part of their care.

- Are you required to purchase a special brace only fabricated by that therapist or required to attend an expensive multi-day program? These requirements should cause you to pause and ask more questions. Research any brace recommended by any practitioner first. Remember, the soft brace has very poor results in the research.

- A full exam should be given as previously outlined and any X-ray or other images must be examined.

- The sagittal (front-to-back curves) plane should be addressed in the program and not just the lateral (side-to-side) curves.

- Breathing is an integral part of any Schroth-based program and should be included.

- ADLs (activities of daily living) should be addressed to emphasize good habits with sitting, standing, walking, etc. to support any exercise program so as not to "un-do" the good work. These corrections are incredibly valuable to give spine support all day and not just during exercises. Hours of "good habits" are incredible for supporting any program.

- If the curves are larger (over 60-80º), the exercises may be given in a more lying down environment to reduce gravity on the spine and its large curves.

- If the curves are not as large - more powerful exercises may be given in the upright position to implement balance, coordination and gravity on the spine as well as activate the muscles against gravity.

- Using too many props, toys, or tools can make your home program unrealistic and add a roadblock to success.

- Be aware of unrealistic promises or time-based goals.

- Is the program that is created for you written down for home reference or other support materials given?

- Were your work, exercise, or sports taken into consideration during the program creation?

15. PAIN RELIEF

Approximately one-quarter of patients with adolescent idiopathic scoliosis present with back pain. Back pain is common in the general population, thus making studies evaluating back pain, specifically in scoliosis, difficult. I have heard it said by those in the medical community that scoliosis doesn't cause pain but those of us who have scoliosis know the truth. It does.

Topical Pain Relief

Powerful analgesic terpenes are aromatic compounds extracted from plants such as camphor, mint (menthol), eucalyptus, clove, tea tree, peppermint and other essential oils that create a cooling or heating sensation when applied to the skin. They deliver soothing relief for muscle and joint pain by interrupting pain signals in the skin's sensory receptors with a heating or cooling sensation. They are so powerful that over-the-counter pharmaceutical manufacturers use them as active ingredients in their topical remedies blended with soothing emollient bases because they know they work. Most topical analgesic products use cheap, synthetic ingredients for their base, including benzyl alcohol, cetyl alcohol, diglycol stearate, glycerol monostearate, etc. Look for a formulation made with natural emollients including jojoba seed oil, beeswax, Shea butter, cottonseed oil and other plant-based extracts.

CBD

CBD stands for cannabidiol, a natural chemical found in the cannabis Sativa plant, more commonly known as marijuana or hemp. CBD does NOT contain THC (tetrahydrocannabinol), the psychoactive ingredient in marijuana that makes you feel high. CBD or cannabis-based products can be topical or ingested and are used as natural remedies for chronic pain, anxiety, insomnia and other conditions. You can find CBD in beauty products, foods, drinks, pills and pet products even though the FDA hasn't approved CDB for these uses. Due to this, there may be variations in product quality and dosage. It is strongly suggested that you talk to your doctor about CDB before use.

CBD activates the molecules that promote a healthy skin barrier since it contains antioxidants that protect the skin from free radicals and oxidative stress on the skin. It contains two essential fatty acids, omega-3 and omega-6, which are thought to support the healthy function of skin, bones and joints. For this reason, CBD is becoming an increasingly popular ingredient in topical formulations.

Is it scientifically proven? At the time of publishing, the FDA has approved only Epidiolex, a prescription drug used to treat some forms of childhood epilepsy (Dravet syndrome and Lennox-Gastaut syndrome).

Are there any health risks associated with CBD? Some potential side effects of CBD are nausea, fatigue and irritability. CBD may have drug interactions with a lot of common medications such as pain medications, psychiatric medications, blood thinners and antihistamines. You must consult with your doctor to review your medications before using CBD. Some CBD products may contain harmful impurities (like pesticides and bacteria). Pregnant and breastfeeding women should not use CBD products.

Is CBD regulated? CBD products are not regulated or evaluated by any government agency.

Will CBD show up on a drug test? CBD shouldnot show up on a drug test unless it contains some THC.

Not sure about CBD? Reach out to your doctor.

Mattress

What works best for you will vary on a case-by-case basis. Many people find that sleeping on a high-quality mattress with medium firmness is ideal for those suffering from scoliosis.

It is not a good idea to sleep on your stomach, as this causes additional rotational stress on both the neck and spine. Back sleeping tends to create the least amount of stress on scoliosis curves but most will need a pillow under the knees or a wedge under large curve areas to get comfortable.

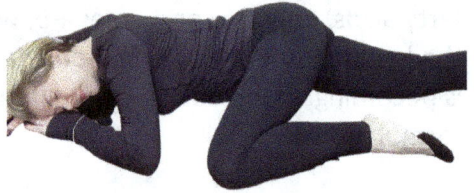

You may wish to use a body pillow between the knees and ankles to support the hips, shoulders and spine while you sleep on your side.

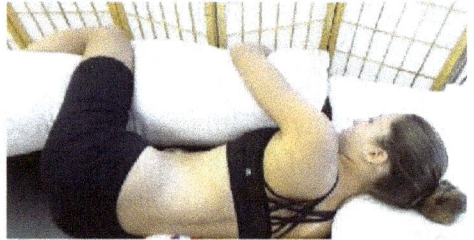

Work with a physical therapist, a Schroth therapist, or other practitioners to find the best pillow options for your specific curve as each case is unique and getting it right is very important. After all, hours of your life are spent sleeping so the ergonomics of your sleeping position and the quality of your sleep matter! Chapter 13 "Nutrition" discussed Melatonin which is a hormone released by the brain and is associated with the wake-sleep cycle among other things and can affect growth if it is too low. How? Melatonin is released during deep sleep which is when human growth hormone is secreted. So, if melatonin is properly being released during sleep, proper growth is better supported. To achieve this, a

186

normal sleep schedule should be implemented and the room should be dark to allow the proper release of melatonin by the brain. Supplementing with melatonin should be done only when a test has been made to determine that your levels are low. It is always best to use it under medical supervision.

Water
It is important to support the discs between the vertebrae. The center of each disc is composed primarily of water. To keep the discs healthy, you want to drink a 1/2 ounce of water per pound of body weight. So, someone who weighs 100 lbs., needs to drink about 50 ounces of water per day, which is roughly equivalent to 4 12-ounce bottles a day. Just do your best!

Drugs/Over the Counter and Prescription
It is always check with your doctor before taking any over-the-counter pain reliever to be sure it is appropriate for you and won't have any interactions with any other medication that you may be taking. If an opioid pain medication is used, it should have instructions for how to gradually wean off the medication over a few weeks. If no specific instructions are given, ask the surgeon and/or pharmacist for recommendations. Proper medication management is important. Over or under-medicating each has its risks. Be alert for allergies if taking a new medication and remember, pain is counterproductive to healing so follow your instructions carefully. I discussed CBD usage for pain and that pain can be an indicator of infection or another serious medical issue. Always check with your doctor if severe or chronic pain develops.

Physical Therapy
PT may be prescribed by your doctor for a scoliosis condition and usually involves exercises that support the core, the spinal muscles and balance activities which are all very beneficial for scoliosis. Unfortunately, most PTs aren't trained in scoliosis-

specific postural exercises and the therapy likely won't be specific to the weaker muscle groups or work asymmetrically. You should ask your PT if he or she has specific scoliosis skills or training before venturing into treatment. You could also ask your doctor for a referral to a Schroth exercise specialist instead and always check with your insurance first. Not all physical therapists are the same or have the same training. Many get extra specialized training for scoliosis and will be an asset to you and should become part of your team.

Chiropractic
Chiropractic care is frequently discouraged by the medical community in general and for a scoliosis condition specifically. This is truly unfortunate as chiropractic care administered by a knowledgeable practitioner can substantially relieve pain and make life much more comfortable. Unfortunately, most chiropractors aren't trained in scoliosis care or scoliosis-specific postural exercises. I was not trained in scoliosis care and I went to a prestigious chiropractic college. Scoliosis training must be taken as a post-graduate course for any practitioner. You should ask your chiropractor if he or she has specific scoliosis skills or training before venturing into treatment. Virtually no formal research exists documenting chiropractic manual manipulation having effectiveness in managing, improving, or "curing" scoliosis, although there are many anecdotal reports of success. Patients should be referred to a spinal orthopedist or neurosurgeon if the scoliosis curves keep increasing. I relied on chiropractic as a pain reliever only and strongly believe it is an appropriate part of any scoliosis care however it should be combined with scoliosis-specific postural exercises and bracing when indicated. Beware of chiropractors who make big promises about scoliosis improvement.

Massage

Massage can relieve pain by softening tight muscles, increasing blood flow to the muscles and tissues, releasing the membranes that wrap around the muscles, enhancing mobility and promoting better sleep which can decrease inflammation that causes pain. Never allow a massage therapist to perform skeletal adjustments unless he or she is trained to do so. The only concern I have with relying on massage for pain management is that the tight muscles on the outside areas of the curves of a scoliosis (the convex side) are doing a tough job of trying to stabilize a curve from bending more into its concavity. By releasing these muscles the support system is now compromised and will create a vicious cycle of scoliosis muscular imbalance.

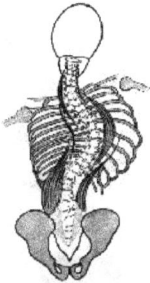

Convexity (outer edge of curve)
) = over extended muscles with decreased muscle contractive capacity and expanded ribs "TIGHT"

Concavity (inner edge of curve)
(= short atrophied muscles and closed ribs, airspace and lungs. "WEAK"

It is so important to be working on the elongation, expansion and activation of the muscles inside the concavity of a curve. The goal is to create more symmetry and balance in the system, so although I used massage for years to manage my pain, I never truly got lasting relief until I began the work of strengthening the weaker muscles too. I recommend that massage work be combined with a program of scoliosis-specific exercises to make sure that imbalances aren't allowed to continue the cycle of weakness and tight muscles.

With my scoliosis you can see the tight muscles on my right side as the curve bends to the right

The weaker spot on the left inside the curve concavity.

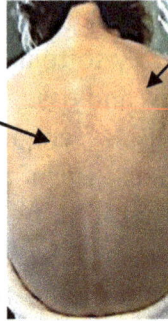

I spent years trying to release the right side only to create more imbalance around my curve.

Once I started working the left side, the right side became much less painful!

Traction

In the Schroth method, there are a few exercises that focus on tractioning the spine and have provided excellent pain relief for myself and my patients. It can be as simple as pulling away from a kitchen sink and sitting into a "chair" position or hanging from a pull-up bar. The hands and shoulders may not enjoy the hanging exercises so there are other options.

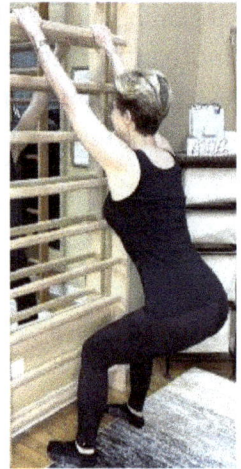

Specs to Build Stall Bars

Two bars made from solid wood (Ash wood is suggested). Upright poles spaced 39" apart, and 92" tall. 18 ladder rungs: 1 1/2" diameter, spaced 5" apart. Mirror behind it.

Inversion

I use an inversion table (hanging upside down) for myself and for my patients and the results are truly amazing.

Inversion has been used for health benefits since ancient times. In 3000 BC humans used inversion as depicted in drawings discovered by archaeologists. In 400 B.C.E., the father of medicine, Hippocrates, hung people on a ladder with ropes and

190

pulleys in an effort to stretch patients and relieve their ailments. In modern times a home use inversion traction table is an adjustable platform that allows positioning in an upright or inverted position to allow variable intensity traction.

Inversion therapy or zero gravity helps:

- Back pain
- Compression on discs
- Nerve pain
- Muscle pain
- Circulation
- Lymph drainage
- Relaxation of muscles
- Mobility of the spine
- Joint mobility
- Flexibility

It creates stretching of paraspinal vertebral muscles and ligaments and creates decompression of intervertebral discs and spinal nerves. Medical studies support that inversion therapy can reduce pain and the need for surgical intervention and people with herniated discs, spinal stenosis, sciatica and other back problems.

Most inversion units have little to no instructions included so get professional instruction and always follow doctor's orders regarding your health before attempting. Here are the instructions I provide my patients:

Inversion can relieve stress, elongate the spine, muscles and discs and aid the body's circulatory system. While securely strapped onto the inversion table, you tilt yourself upside down to your desired degree. Once there, you can stretch or perform some breathing without any pressure being placed on your spine. Of course, simply hanging upside down and relaxing is always an option. Always follow doctor's orders regarding your health before attempting. It is NOT advised with:

Hiatus Hernia / Glaucoma / High Blood Pressure (Hypertension) / Dizziness / Bone weakness (osteoporosis, recent unhealed fractures, pins, artificial hip joints or other orthopedic surgical implant or fusion / Cardiovascular insufficiencies in the limbs / After head injury / Poorly coordinated / Fainting spells / Acute spinal injury / Disoriented if upside down / Weak or frail / Retinal detachment / Cerebral sclerosis / Recent stroke or transient ischemic attack / Heart and circulatory disorders for which you are being treated / Acutely swollen joints / Chronic sinusitis / Motion sickness or inner ear disorders...Or any other medical condition that may be made more severe by an elevation of blood pressure or intracranial pressure.

Step 1: Adjust the inversion table to your height. Your head should rest comfortably on the table and not hang over the edge. Read the directions carefully when adjusting your table since each manufacturer may use different mechanics.
Step 2: Decide the degree to which you want to invert. Begin at 45º or less. Increase the inversion gradually as you acclimate to being upside down. Many inversion tables come with a safety strap or stopper that allows you to choose your inversion degree; adjust to your preference. More is NOT better! A slight traction angle is plenty to feel the effects.

Step 3: Stand with your back against the table and place your feet in the footrests. Follow your table's directions for securing your feet. Lean back to rotate the table to slowly invert. Wear Ugg® type boots if your ankles get sore.

Step 4: Breathe deeply as you hang upside down and relax. Stay inverted for as long as you are comfortable. Beginners may find it disconcerting to be upside down at first; consider **inverting for just two to three minutes to start** and gradually work your way up to 10 minutes as you become more comfortable if you are doing this daily. If you take a break of more than a few days start at 2-3 minutes again and work back up. **DO NOT overdo it!!!!!!**

Step 5: Reach your arms up behind your head so that your arms are straight and your spine is elongated. Hold the stretch for as long as you feel comfortable. Aim for at least 30 to 60 seconds. I find it helpful to "wiggle" to create the best stretch as my back gets a bit stuck to the table and needs to be freed up.

Step 6: Pull yourself up with the handles when you are ready to return to an upright position. Return back up **very slowly** to avoid feeling dizzy. I like to slowly roll up and fold forward to stretch my hamstrings before unlocking the ankles. Wait until you feel steady before unlocking the footrests and stepping out of the inversion table.

Wedging
In the Schroth method, we use wedges under the scoliotic curves to "unwind" the spine and allow it to relax as well as create some curve correction by passively de-rotating the rotations in the spine. Your scoliosis practitioner/therapist may have given you specific wedges or pillows to use with your specific scoliosis. This is different for each person so there is no value in following a generic guide that was not prescribed to YOU. Be sure to follow your wedge instructions carefully and add them to your daily life such as your workouts, resting, or sleeping. Wedging properly can reduce pain significantly and works very well for my patients.

Breathing Exercises
As done in Chapter 12 "Exercise and Scoliosis," breathing can open the compressed ribcage, oxygenate, lengthen, strengthen the muscles and relieve pain. Even if it is as simple as adding a deep breath during the workday or commute, it is so useful in reducing pain. This takes us to our next topic....

Daily Habits
While the scoliosis-specific postural exercise programs are remarkable as are all of the other pain relief techniques, nothing can serve you better than taking care of your daily habits which add up to many hours of your day. If you are working hard on your program and doing everything you can but have a day riddled with bad habits, you are not going to make as much progress. It is important to know how to sit, stand, walk and even sleep with proper body mechanics for your scoliosis. If you are working with a therapist make sure you are given activities of daily living (ADLs) to assist you. Simply leaning onto a curve while sitting for many hours or standing and jutting out a hip that is already shifted due to scoliosis can set you back and be contributing to curve progression and or pain. In my Schroth practice, these issues are addressed first. I even consider what sports, hobbies and job tasks can be modified to help the daily support of a curvature. Adding the Schroth breath to your daily corrective postures and exercise programs or sports go a long way in shutting down pain.

Brace Pain
While a brace is not the most comfortable experience, it should never be painful or cause any sores or issues. If you are concerned with any discomfort wearing your brace you should consult your orthotist for help and a possible brace adjustment. Almost no brace is perfect the first time you wear it, it needs to be customized and fine-tuned in the beginning and as the curve

changes, so will the brace need to be modified. More padding may be added, rough spots shaved down or straps changed. As the curve is corrected by the brace the brace and even the SSPE plan you are on will need to change to follow your progress. This is an evolving process, be patient and flexible as your therapists fine-tune your scoliosis tools with you.

Nutrition
As stated in Chapter 13 "Nutrition," inflammation plays a very big role in pain management. Avoiding foods that trigger inflammation will only help your overall well-being.

Heat/Ice
Always consult with your healthcare professional when applying heat or ice either when you are in pain, or recovering from an injury or surgery. Your particular case may be special and require specific instructions. Be careful not to overuse either heat or ice. It is possible to burn your skin with heat and even with ice.

Journaling
Patients have reported that it helps to distract themselves with journaling or other activities to get their mind off of any pain they are experiencing.

EMDR Therapy
Eye movement desensitization and reprocessing (EMDR) therapy is a mental health treatment technique. This method involves moving your eyes a specific way while you process traumatic memories. EMDR's goal is to help you heal from trauma or other distressing life experiences. Compared to other therapy methods, EMDR is relatively new. The first clinical trial investigating EMDR was in 1989. Dozens of clinical trials since EMDR's development show this technique is effective and can help a person faster than many other methods. EMDR can help people with a wide range of

mental health conditions. Adolescents, teenagers and adults of all ages can benefit from this treatment. Some healthcare providers also specialize in EMDR for children.

EMDR therapy does not require talking in detail about a distressing issue. EMDR instead focuses on changing the emotions, thoughts or behaviors that result from a distressing experience (trauma). This allows your brain to resume a natural healing process. This has therapy can also be useful during bracing, pre or post-surgery, or to help a child if they are being bullied at school.

https://www.emdr.com/

16. PSYCHOLOGY OF SCOLIOSIS

When first diagnosed with scoliosis regardless of age, one may feel overwhelmed, embarrassed, different from others, or "deformed". Feelings of being different and standing out are extraordinarily difficult for youngsters, especially females.

Whether you are the parent or patient it can quickly become a situation where you can feel helpless and frustrated and not know what happens next or whom to listen to. It's time to build your team and start the steps to learn more. I hope this book helps you to build your team and make informed choices. Learn the tools and explore the options. Knowledge is power.

Two types of personalities may react to scoliosis differently
The introverted person with social inhibitions, a preference for staying alone and physical shyness will avoid situations where people can see their bodies and will construct ways to function as normally as possible while hiding the curvature. Some of these coping skills may cause more pain or curve progression due to postural issues such as creating a protective shell both mentally and physically. These personality types likely have more curve progression and it will take extra effort and diligence to treat the scoliosis. A passive "victim mentality" is easily adopted and the paralysis of doing nothing either by the parent or the patient is the worst choice one can make.

The opposite type of patient is the one who is determined to succeed in dealing with their condition. This often translates into self-guided physical activity or physical therapy and possibly trying too hard. Over-gripping and overworking can activate stronger muscle groups and create more pain. Trying to keep control over the situation can cause undue stress and overwork or overzealous treatment.

Acceptance of scoliosis and recognizing that it makes you unique is a positive place to start. Be aware of what you are experiencing physically and mentally and try not to judge your feelings. Try simply to observe.

An important note for parents:
Scoliosis has been found to be a risk factor for psychosocial issues and health-compromising behavior. Speak with your child and get them some help if they need it. Keep open lines of communication and monitor their mental wellness.

Support Groups
Ask your orthotist, doctor, or therapist, or do your own internet search for options. I have compiled a list in the next chapter, "Resources". Social media outlets now have thousands of people of all ages posting about their experiences with their scoliosis.

There have been many cases where people have an emotional or physical response during treatment. There have been cases of reacting to breath work, to an exercise, to being placed into a new posture position during therapy, or even just wearing the brace. Sometimes these reactions are feelings of being tearful, dizzy, or nauseous. This is normal so it is alright to stop or slow down, take a breath and try again. If the feeling continues you should talk to your practitioner or orthotist.

As a practitioner, I stop and let my patient relax. I try to offer supportive dialogue or leave them alone for a minute. I offer them water, tissues and a private place to gather themselves or talk for a minute. Just listen, be understanding and be supportive. It will pass. The bonding between patient and therapist is important, there needs to be trust between you and your therapist along this journey.

Many people have deep feelings and emotional issues surrounding their scoliosis. Adults may have been bullied or shamed as children, subjected to difficult scoliosis braces that were traumatizing and didn't work well or they weren't compliant and now have regrets. Some get emotional discussing it and do NOT want to see their X-rays or even a drawing of the curves to understand them. If this is you or your child, ask your doctor or therapist to use other props to convey the information you need in a new way to see your curve and work on it. It is your body and you deserve to be treated in a way that makes you most comfortable.

Exercise or Bracing Stress
Not everybody is happy to have to focus on time to do therapy, exercise, or wear a brace. It's important to confront this stress and get help from your practitioner, family therapist and reach out to support groups to communicate with others who are going through the same journey. Parents can get into a battle with their child regarding the wearing of the brace or the exercise routines. If a child is extraordinarily stressed by exercise, focus on the brace. If the brace is the main issue, discuss this with your orthotist and go back to reading Chapter 9 "Bracing".

Therapist or Parent Strategies
"De-pathologize" and normalize the situation - scoliosis is very common!

Helpful Support Tips For Family and Therapists
* Children should stay involved in sports and activities.

- Give your child a break from the brace or exercises for a sleepover, a vacation, or a special event.

- Hug your child every day.

- Talk to other parents.

- Communicate with your child. Most importantly, listen to their thoughts and concerns.

- Using terms like "empty space", "inside of the curve", "hollow areas" and rotations instead of using terms like "hump", "caved-in area", deformity and even "bump" which can be a trigger word for some and sound negative.

- Keep it light-hearted, supportive and positive.

- Use basic language. Fancy anatomy terms can alienate or even trigger memories of bad medical experiences.

- Be a coach, be part of the team.

- Give your child helpful information: Facebook groups, books, videos, etc.

- Teach your child some basic anatomy so that they have tools to understand and be active in their program.

- Therapists should teach ADLs (activities of daily living) to support the person in their life outside of the exercise routines and outside of the clinic.

Helpful Support Tips From Other Teens:

- Talk to others who have scoliosis, there are thousands out there!

- You can do this - you are tough.

- Your brace is a part of you now - name it and em-brace it!

- Let your friends in on what is going on with you.

- Start a journal or blog or vlog of your journey.

- Go shopping for new clothes that cover the brace.
- It's just like braces on your teeth, it's so temporary.

Please read this contribution from Lauren Higginson the founder of Higgy Bears (higgybears.com). Higgy Bears creates custom doll braces to match your brace in all shapes and colors. It is also a website with many other accessories and a robust support resource for all things scoliosis related.

Lauren Higginson contributes the following: "Scoliosis is hard. It is hard physically and it is hard emotionally. Surgeons, physical therapists and orthotists have the physical side covered, but who helps your child through this emotionally? That's where I come in! Hi, My name is Lauren Higginson and I am the founder of Higgy Bears. I was diagnosed with scoliosis when I was thirteen and never knew anyone else 'like me' growing up. I felt incredibly alone and cried myself to sleep most nights. As an adult, I wanted to find a way to keep other kids from feeling the way I did, so I created Higgy Bears. Higgy Bears are special little friends that go through the same treatment as your child or teen, just in bear form. I hand-make mini back braces for the bears to wear and sew rods in their backs for patients, like me, that have had spinal fusion surgery. They are a little friend where one did not exist. Kids take their Higgy Bears with them to that scary first appointment and cuddle up with them at night. They truly help make scoliosis more 'bear-able' for kids. In addition to making Higgy Bears, I also run several support programs to connect kids. Higgy Bears are so very helpful, but if your child can meet another child going through the same thing, it will make an even bigger difference. I host ScoliZoom meetings every month for kids, tweens, teens and parents. It is a wonderful opportunity for kids to come together virtually and support one another. We have a blast. In the kid's group, we play fun scoliosis-themed games and laugh the entire time. The kids love to share what pattern they have on their brace and are so excited when another kid has the same pattern. The tweens and teens love to share their stories and support and encourage one another. They share lots of wonderful bracing, fashion and surgery tips. They enjoy getting to see and talk to other kids that are going through the same thing. The kids even set up Kids Messenger Groups and chat groups so they can stay in contact with one another outside of ScoliZooms. I have enjoyed getting to know the kids and it is so heartwarming to see them support one another. One of the teen girls refused to wear her brace before she joined ScoliZooms. The girls rallied around her and encouraged her every day to wear her brace. She now wears her brace proudly and joins every meeting so she can pay it forward and help others. Being able to visually see that other kids have scoliosis makes such a huge difference.

I highly recommend getting your kid or teen involved in ScoliZooms. You can view the most current schedule on the ScoliZoom tab at higgybears.com".

"Scoliosis is hard on everyone, but I've found that it's especially hard on boys. There isn't much support out there for boys, which makes them feel even more alone. I created ScoliBoys to help boys and their parents. Hundreds of families have joined my ScoliBoys Support Group on Facebook so they can connect and support one another. I would love for you to join if you are on Facebook. The group name is, 'ScoliBoys Scoliosis Support Group for Boys with Scoliosis and Their Parents.' I also highly recommend the Scolios-us Mentor Program. Teens volunteer as mentors and encourage kids and teens that join as mentees. They connect through text, video chat, or phone. It's a one-on-one approach compared to the group atmosphere of ScoliZooms. The teens make such a huge difference to the patients they mentor. You can learn more about this wonderful mentor program by visiting www.bracingforscoliosus.org.

202

"Scoliosis doesn't just affect the child or teen living with the condition. It's hard on parents, too. Just like the kids, you also need support. There are so many wonderful Scoliosis Facebook Groups for parents. There are thousands of parents out there going through the same thing that you are that would love to help and support you. Trust me, parents are the best resource. They've encountered the same problems and have the very best tips. The scoliosis community is so incredibly supportive. I highly recommend you reach out and get involved.

"In addition to the support programs, I love to run fun contests for the kids to get involved in. Be sure to follow Higgy Bears on Facebook and Instagram for the latest updates! One of the programs that kids love the most is my Higgy Bears Ambassador Program. Kids will set up fundraisers to be able to purchase several Higgy Bears. When their fundraiser is complete, they get to pick out what animals and braces they would like. I then make everything and send all the Higgy Animals directly to them. Your child or teen then takes the Higgy Bears into their local clinic or hospital to donate. It gives the kids such a huge sense of pride and makes them so happy by being able to give back and help other kids. Nearly ten thousand Higgy Bears have been donated by kids through this program. To learn more, please visit the 'How to Help' tab on my website or email me for more information.

"As you can see, your family is not alone. I would love for you to get involved in the programs that I run. If you have any questions, or if there is anything I can do to help you, please do not hesitate to reach out to me at lauren@higgybears.com. Always remember, we may be bent, but we are not broken!"

17. RESOURCES

SHOP:
To view a curated shop of items I recommend for my patients.
http://www.scoliosiscoach.com/shop.html

Custom doll and teddy bear braces, T-shirts, bracelets, journals, and more. https://higgybears.com/shop

Clothes:

- The "Scoliosis Tank" on Etsy has a flap to cover brace edges under the arm.
- www.Tillys.com Torso "Sock" – with or without flap
- http://royalknit.com/products/torso-socks/
- http://www.bostonbrace.com/content/accessories.asp
- Sugar Lips (No underarm flap)
- SmartKnitKIDS Seamless or compression
- Uniqlo™
- EmBraced in Comfort
- Singlosport
- DiabeticSock
- The Boston T (with armpit flap) is a protective body sock made of CoolMax™/Lycra, with an antibacterial fiber
- BraceBuddies
- Rosette seamless shirts
- Under Armour™ seamless shirts
- For Boys: Jockey™ Seam-Free Crew, Fun and Function Tees, Sierra Trading Post T-shirt

- http://scoliosisliving.blogspot.com/2014/04/what-to-wear-under-your-scoliosis-brace.html

Higgy Bears & Scolios-us Clothing Tips From Kids
"If you feel like you want to hide your brace, you can wear your pants/shorts over your brace, then wear spandex or bike shorts under the brace. This way if your shirt comes up you see regular pants. Just make sure you keep an eye on your pants, you can't feel them if they fall down." - Claire

"Leggings, leggings, leggings!! If you don't wear a uniform" - Holly

"Everything oversized (tees, hoodies) and leggings or sweatpants are lifesavers" - Illiana

"Wear a T one size down from your regular size under your school blouse/shirt. You could also seek permission from your school to wear your blouse as a tunic instead of tucked in for your comfort." - Ann

Support
Scoliosis can be challenging for anybody but it also can be hard on the family. This is where social media can be a gold mine. There are so many amazing groups that offer support not only from medical professionals but parents, kids and other people going through exactly what you are.

Facebook Groups - A List Curated by Lauren Higginson:
- Scoliosis Support Group for Teens, Tweens, and Parents
- Mothers of Children with Scoliosis
- Parents of Kids with Juvenile Scoliosis
- ScoliBoys Support Group

- Embraced Scoliosis Support Group for Parents
- Dr. Derek Lee's Ultimate Guide to Navigating Scoliosis Treatment/Research
- Scoliosis Support Group Girls Aged 8-12
- Early Onset Juvenile Scoliosis Support Group
- Scoliosis Support Group
- Infantile Scoliosis
- Early Onset Scoliosis & Mehta Casting
- Scoliosis Tethering (VBT & ASC) Support group specifically for parents and patients interested in learning about surgery.

Websites

- www.bracingforscoliosus.org A mentor program and resource center.
- Scoliosis & Spine Online Learning (SSOL) https://www.scoliosisandspineonlinelearning.com A website with information and webinars from top scoliosis professionals across the world.
- www.settingscoliosisstraight.org Setting Scoliosis Straight
- www.aaos.org American Academy of Orthopedic Surgeons
- www.srs.org Scoliosis Research Society
- www.posna.org Pediatric Orthopedic Society of North America www.scoliosis.org National Scoliosis Foundation
- www.scoliosis-assoc.org The Scoliosis Association
- www.kidshealth.org/scoliosis Kids Health

- Curvy Girls is one of the largest organizations supporting children with a forum, events, store, etc.
- SupportGroups.com
- A Dutch language website in the Netherlands www.Scoliose.nl
- In the UK The Scoliosis Association www.sauk.org.uk
- HiggyBears.com has a comprehensive toolbox to assist families, girls and boys with Zoom groups, conventions, clothing and more.

Blogs

- https://scoliosissiblings.wordpress.com/
- www.scoliosisnutty.blogspot.com - A cute little blog on scoliosis.
- scoliosis-braceyourself.blogspot.com - Another blog about scoliosis
- scoliosisliving.blogspot.com - A blog about a family going through the struggles of Scoliosis.

Anatomy Digital Portals

- Primal Pictures
- www.BooksOfDiscovery.com
- AnatomyZone - YouTube channel by Dr. Souza and Dr. Hurley
- TeachMeAnatomy - A visual anatomy encyclopedia.
- BioDigital - 3-D interactive models.
- InnerBody - Interactive learning tool with 3D images.
- BodyMaps - Explore the human body in 3-D.
- Get Body Smart - An eBook of human anatomy and physiology.

- Muscle Atlas - UW Department of Radiology
- The Visible Human Project - Complete 3D male and female human bodies. National Library of Medicine.
- Workshop Anatomy for the Internet - A collection of detailed images of human anatomical structures.
- BIODIC: The ultrastructure website - by the Free University of Brussels.
- Gray's Anatomy by Bartleby
- Web Anatomy - by Murray Jensen from the Univ. of Minnesota.
- Anatomy & physiology resources from RM Chute.
- The Whole Brain Atlas from Harvard Medical School.
- Anatomy Models - University of Colorado at Boulder.
- Anatomy & Physiology Animations - Lone Star College.
- Muscle Physiology from the National Skeletal Muscle Research Center at UC San Diego.

Schroth Therapy
To find a Schroth therapist and learn more about Schroth:
https://www.schrothmethod.com/resources-for-child

Schroth Method Exercises for Scoliosis:
https://www.schrothmethod.com

Worldwide Schroth Therapist Directory:
https://www.schrothmethod.com/contact

Schroth-Barcelona Institute:
https://www.schroth-barcelonainstitute.com

Bracing Videos

- https://youtu.be/GkKPNIksFmg
- https://youtu.be/3cxSqsdKo3g

Books

Children's books:

- Exercise - What It Is, What It Does by Carola Trier

Books for Kids/Tweens:

- The Silver Horned Gir,l by Lisa Owens. Highly recommend for both children and teens. Amazing book to help with self-confidence with wearing a back brace or having surgery.
- The Scoliosaurus, by Lauren Amy Davis
- Being Grace: A Story for Children About Scoliosis, by June Hyjek
- Beamer Learns About Scoliosis, by Cindy Chambers
- Cole & The Crooked Flower, by Russell Leggett
- Beautiful Crooked Letter I, by Shae Smith
- Scolios-us Brace Journal, by BracingforScoliosus.org
- Braced, by Alyson Gerber
- Straight Talk with the Curvy Girls, by Theresa E. Mulvaney and Robin Stoltz
- Fighting the Curve: My Battle with Scoliosis, by Haley Guidry
- Harry Scores a Hat Trick With Pawns, Pucks, and Scoliosis, by Mary Mahogany
- Abby's Twin, by Ann M. Martin
- Heaven Sent, by S.J. Morgan
- Deenie, by Judy Blume

- When Life Throws You a Curve, by Elizabeth Golden
- There's an S on My Back, by Mary Mahoney
- Plastic Back, by Anna Rakes

Books for Parents:
- The Emotional Journey of Scoliosis, by Reshmi Pal
- Help, My Daughter Has Scoliosis, by Hilary Lowne
- What Can I Give You, by Mary Mahoney
- No One Else Like Me, by Karla Auerbach
- I Have Scoliosis, Now What, by Erin Myers
- Scoliosis: A Guide for Children & Their Families, by Michael G. Vitale, MD, MPH, and Amber Mizerik, PA-C
- Setting Scoliosis Straight, Digital Handbooks https://www.settingscoliosisstraight.org/patient-handbook/
- Three-Dimensional Treatment for Scoliosis: A Physiotherapeutic Method for Deformities of the Spine, by Christa Lehnert-Schroth
- Schroth Therapy: Advancements in Conservative Scoliosis Treatment, by Weiss, Hans-Rudolf; Lehnert-Schroth, Christa; Moramarco, Marc
- Schroth's Textbook of Scoliosis and Other Spinal Deformities, by Hans-Rudolf Weiss Marc Moramarco, Maksym Borysov, Shu Yan Ng

Anatomy books:
- Fitness Professionals Guide to Musculoskeletal Anatomy and Human Movement, by Golding and Golding
- Atlas of Human Anatomy, by Frank N. Netter

- Anatomy Coloring Book, by Wynn Kapit and Lawrence M. Elson
- Anatomy of Movement, by Blandine C. Germain
- Anatomy of Movement: Exercises, by Blandine C. Germain and Stephen Anderson
- Illustrated Essentials of Musculoskeletal Anatomy, by Sieg and Adams
- Trail Guide to the Body Text Book & Student Workbook from Books of Discovery, by Andrew Biel

Apps
BraceTrack is a great app for your phone that allows you to track the hours you have worn your brace. Apps and thermal brace trackers (iButton) have been shown to increase compliance with brace-wearing!

Physical Therapy
Scolios-Us Physical Therapy & Exercise Information:
https://www.bracingforscoliosus.org/physical-therapy-and-exercise-information

Financial Resources
HealthWell Foundation: When health insurance is not enough, they may help fill the gap by assisting with copays, premiums, deductibles and out-of-pocket expenses.
https://www.healthwellfoundation.org

The Children's Scoliosis Foundation: offers financial aid grants of up to $500 per trip ($750 for international travel) to help support children and their families who are traveling long distances for bracing or surgical treatment for scoliosis.
https://www.childrensscoliosisfoundation.org

United HealthCare Children's Foundation: UHCCF grants can help with medical expenses not covered, or not fully covered, by health insurance. The amount awarded to an individual within a 12-month period is limited to $5,000. Awards to any one individual are limited to a lifetime maximum of $10,000.
https://www.uhccf.org

Mercy Medical Angels: MMA is the largest charitable medical transportation system in the world. It helps with transportation on the ground including gas cards, bus and train tickets and flights flown by volunteer pilots and commercial airlines.
https://www.mercymedical.org

Instagram
Lauren Higginson of Higgy Bears says: "I recommend if your teen is on Instagram to follow several of the teens that have scoliosis accounts. There are so many wonderful girls out there that are giving back and helping others that have scoliosis. There are several that I recommend. I know these girls personally and they would love to help your child or teen in any way possible through their scoliosis journey. Their DMs are always open."

- Izzy (@scoliosis_warrior_2019)
- Alia (@scoliosis_brace_sister)
- Olivia (@olivia.scoliosis)
- Brooke (@scoliosis.brooke)
- Chloe (@_chloe_strong_)
- Hailey (@haileyscoliosis)
- Sarah (@scoli_sarah)
- Ashlyn (@klaus_the_higgy_koala)

- Several Girls (@higgybearsandbraces)
- Haley (@haley_scoliosis12)
- Hayden (@hayden.scoliosis)
- Lucy (@lucysscoliosis)
- Charlee (@scoliosiswarrior_charlee28)

"Don't forget to follow Higgy Bears! (@higgybears) There aren't any boys that have support accounts on Instagram that I know of (which is unfortunate), but there is a huge need! If your scoliosis teen is interested in starting an account for scoliosis boys, please let us know! We would be happy to share and promote it!"

There are several celebrities and influencers with scoliosis that are great role models.

- Martha Hunt (@marthahunt)
- Meredith Martin (@bionic_ballerina)
- Gigi Crouch (@scolerina9247)
- Kyra Condie (@kyra_condie)
- Paige Fraser (@lovingthispaige)
- Julia Carlile (@juliacarlile_xo)
- Princess Eugenie (@princesseugenie)
- Alyson Gerber (@alysongerber)

YouTube Accounts
Search:
- *Back brace fashion*
- *Back brace tips*
- *Scoliosis surgery tips*

- Surgery Tips from Izzy:
  https://www.youtube.com/@izzyann6798
- Malia Jade Brace Fashion Tips:
  https://www.youtube.com/watch?v=CWUxL43Wygw
  https://www.youtube.com/watch?v=eXjwlzA1xyI
- My Back Brace YouTube Channel:
  https://www.youtube.com/@MyBackBrace
- EmBrace The Brace:
  https://www.youtube.com/channel/UChGKOE2e8DYyj-XKnnqdTHQ

Surgery

- Michael G. Vitale, MD, MPH, Columbia Orthopedics Educational Resources
  https://pediatricscoliosissurgery.com/educational-resources/
- Scoliosis: A Guide for Children & Their Families by Michael G. Vitale, MD, MPH and Amber Mizerik, PA-C
- What to Expect - Your Child's Spine Surgery by Michael G. Vitale, MD, MPH

Higgy Bears Surgery Guide
Helpful Items for Hospital Stay

- Electronic accessories
- Long charger for laptop/tablet and headphones
- Parents, don't forget your phone charger!
- Mini personal fan (very helpful!) The best purchase you can make as the medicine might make you hot and nauseous.
- Pen & paper to take notes
- Adult coloring books or other activity books
- Pillow

- Surgery Higgy Bear to help with recovery
- High-calorie snacks for the patient while they are recovering.
- Bring snacks and a water bottle for the caregiver, too.

Clothes
- PJ (tops) that button up or button-up shirts
- Grippy socks for walking in the hallways
- Underwear
- Elastic shorts or pajama pants
- Slip-on tennis shoes
- Warm socks
- Rolling suitcase

Toiletries
- Toothbrush, toothpaste, comb and a brush
- Chapstick as lips get very dry after surgery.
- Pads or menstrual supplies (the stress of the surgery will cause many girls to start their period).

Car Ride Home
Several pillows for the car. It is hard to get comfortable in the car on the way home. Stool to get in and out of the car if needed.

Recovery At Home - Medical & Helpful Items
- Large ice packs (2 of these) and a large heating pad.
- Laxatives - ask your doctor for instructions as pain meds cause constipation.
- Grabber to be able to reach/pick up things.
- Walker - usually supplied by the hospital.

- Water bottle with a non-leaking squirt top or water bottle with bendy straw to drink while lying down in bed.

Bedroom & Living Room
- About 5-7 pillows for the bed
- Wedge pillows or body pillows
- Lift Recliner chair - you can rent these from medical supply
- Zero Gravity Chair
- Bed support arm to help sit up in bed.
- An adjustable bed is great if you have that option.
- Foam mattress toppers can be helpful to keep you comfortable.

Bathroom
- Shower chair and/or shower stool
- Toilet riser with handles
- Non-slip mat for shower
- Handheld shower head
- Hairdresser cape for washing hair (you can sit in a chair and wash hair or use a cape for privacy/and or to keep clothes dry).
- Loofah on a stick for the shower (you will not be able to bend in the shower).
- Long-reach toilet aid (it can be very hard to wipe after surgery without twisting).
- Urinal for boys
- Baby wipes
- Dry shampoo

Clothing

- Athletic shorts
- Loose pants or PJ pants
- More button-up loose shirts
- Front-closure sports bra

Helpful Tips

- Make a schedule with your child in order to squeeze in all of their PT, meds, water, spirometer, walks, chair time, etc.
- Braid long hair before surgery.
- Join Facebook support groups and post any problems you are having. Stay on top of the pain medicine schedule, even in the middle of the night. Incredibly important.
- Walking is very important after surgery. It's hard, but it helps! Start slowly and work up to longer distances. Use a walker, if needed.
- Ask if the hospital has a program for service animals to come and visit.

Please don't feel like you have to get all of the items on this list. Certain items are helpful for some and not needed for others. Parents, don't forget to take care of yourselves during this time, too. This recovery is hard for your child and it will be hard for you, too. The first couple of days is similar to taking care of a newborn at home. You will need to do everything for your child. Sleep when they sleep. Eat nutritious meals to keep your energy up. Be sure to reach out to parents in Facebook groups for support.
Back to School

- Pillow for chair
- Rolling backpack or a friend to carry their things.

- No bus, drive them
- Ask teachers to dismiss them a few minutes early from each class so as not to be rushed in the hallway.
- Ask if they can still "be on the team" for their sports activities even if they are not playing this season.

Sharing Your Scoliosis with Classmates

The wonderful ladies at Scolios-us put together a PowerPoint presentation kids can present to their class about scoliosis. I've found that teaching classmates about scoliosis and having your child explain to his/her class why he/she needs to wear a scoliosis brace or have surgery is especially helpful for elementary students.

https://www.bracingforscoliosus.org/presentations-for-warriors-heading-back-to-school/

"My daughter (7) starts school on Monday. Got the brace 2 weeks ago. We are planning to have a Q&A session with her class. Met with the school nurse today to coordinate her accommodations. My hope is that the other kiddos will be curious and open to "embracing" this change." - Marilyn

"Just try to be as open as possible. Let the questions come, as curiosity is powerful. People will stare less if they have knowledge. For me personally, my teacher let me go in front of the class, talk about it and then take questions. Never assume that when a person comments on your brace, it's always something negative or that they're being rude to you. Most of the time, people are just curious and have never seen a brace before! Use this as an opportunity to maybe educate them a little! I've had a ton of girls coming up to me and asking about my brace and a few of them (once I explained everything) even discovered they had scoliosis too!" - Callista

504 Plans for School

504 plans are designed to ensure your child receives needed accommodations at school. Definitely look into this if the school is not being helpful with what your child needs. Examples of accommodations in 504 plans include:

- Preferential seating
- Extended time on tests and assignments
- Reduced homework or classwork
- Verbal, visual or technological aids
- Modified textbook or audio-video materials
- Behavior management support
- Adjusted class schedules or grading
- Verbal testing
- Excused lateness, absence, or missed classwork
- To learn more about this program and others https://www.cta.org/understanding-504-plans

How 504 plans can help scoliosis patients
"We asked for a top locker, made sure she had a chair with a back, the ability to stand anytime as needed, extra books for home or to leave in the classroom, the ability to leave class early if needed to get stuff from locker and instrument if needed, ability to go to the nurse anytime. This was stuff right after her surgery but we kept it and still have it 4 years later."

"We requested one with a doctor's note in hand. Our doctor put in some recommendations in the note (air conditioning, brace breaks, using restrooms in nurses' offices, options for chairs, set of materials for home, etc). Once the school had the note, the school psychologist observed Paige in class. We had the 504 meeting and she was found eligible. Paige goes to the nurse to take her brace off for PE and recess. The nurse holds the brace in her office when she is not wearing it." - Melissa

"Stretch breaks!! My daughter is in middle school now, but even in elementary, the schools have been very good at allowing her to just stand up next to her desk and stretch for a minute." - Tennille

"I'm a school psychologist with scoliosis and a parent of 3. 504 plans have different criteria in different states/counties. In Florida and in my district, a parent needs to present a letter from a doctor with a diagnosis to the school. The parent can request a 504 meeting and this meeting will consist of a team of professionals." - Lauren

Other Tips from Kids and Parents
Seating: "The hard plastic chairs stink and can be super uncomfortable. Ask your teachers for a different chair. In past years, they've given me the soft office chairs which are so helpful!" "You can make a little pad to make the chairs more comfortable (it helped me more when I didn't have my brace but it could be helpful with a brace.)"

"Make sure to talk to your teachers to get some extra time to stretch during class if you need to because wearing a brace and sitting all day can make your back really stiff and sore." - Karen

"Offer to run papers for the teacher so you can get up and walk around!" - Lily

"For surgery patients: bring a pillow (whatever softness or firmness is best for you!) to help support your back, most chairs are horrible after surgery."- Madelynn

"I like a backpack with thicker, more padded straps so they don't pinch my skin (between your brace and backpack.)." - Teagan

"My daughter used a rolling backpack when she wore a brace. We made sure to put it in her 504 plan because some schools don't allow rolling backpacks." - Claire

"When I was bracing I used a smaller tote bag that I could just carry by hand instead of putting all the weight on my shoulders." - Madelynn

"A Higgy Bear Brace Bag is a great way to store your brace and keep it covered if you have to take it off for gym or sports."- Alex

"If you need help carrying books, ask a friend whom you trust!" - Kat

"Ask for an extra set of books to keep at home." - Hailey

"At my daughter's middle school, they had top lockers and bottom lockers. We always made sure she got a top locker, so she wouldn't need to squat. And she used a rolling backpack. She also got a second copy of all of her textbooks, so she wouldn't have to carry them in her backpack." - Kymberly

"I played sports when I had two curves over 50 degrees. Something that helped me was taking my medicine right before practice/games. Definitely helped with the pain. Extra stretching helped me so much, too! Yoga can help as well!" - Vickie

"Doctor's note!!! Neither my middle school or high school accepted parent notes, so just make sure you have a doctor's note that specifically says things you can't do or says you can decide what you feel comfortable with. Communication with the teacher,

PE teacher and nurse about getting a few minutes before and after PE to take off and put back on the brace. I will encourage our school nurse to remind my daughter to tighten it up!" - Juliette "Talk to your school nurse! I used to always feel nervous going to the bathroom in my brace at school and she gladly let me use hers anytime! Best decision I've made so far!" - Alyssa

"I would highly recommend either the person in the brace or a parent talking to a teacher/teachers about any difficulties with the brace. I had to get my brace in September last year so I told my teacher about my situation and said I would need a seat in the back of the class so I could stand when needed when my back got sore and I also needed more time in the bathroom (it took me about 10 minutes for the first month I had it) so communication is key!!" - Maddie

"Bus seats are hard on kids! See how long their route is. Sometimes transportation can have your student on a shorter route if they need it. Transportation, the buses, are always happy to try to help! Just call and ask! Also, if they have had surgery recently, see if the transportation will allow your child to ride the small bus. They can pick up at the house and shorter ride. Seating pad for longer rides if that is needed." - Michele

"For even more school tips, search in the Facebook Support Groups or ask the question yourself. There are thousands of parents out there that have been through the same thing you are and would be happy to help you and your child". - Annie

Higgy Bears Ambassador Program
"Join dozens of kids all over the world that have started Higgy Bear Fundraisers! Kids can fundraise any way they would like and when their fundraiser is complete, they get to pick out all of the animals they would like. Higgy Bears will send the dolls directly to

your child and they can personally take them into their hospital or clinic to donate. This is a great volunteer opportunity for your child. Kids and teens really enjoy giving back and helping other kids. Please visit higgybears.com and click on how to help for more information or send us an email".

Dr. Stevens' Video Portals

- YouTube Scoliosis Coach
- YouTube Pilates Sports Center
- https://vimeo.com/scoliosiscoach
- Membership Portal Scoliosis Coach

Pilates Membership Video Portals (not scoliosis related)

- Membership Portal Pilates Sports Center
- https://vimeo.com/pilatessportscenter

Pilates Digital Shop (not scoliosis related) Digital Downloads Shop

Social
Connect with me to stay motivated and informed
@ScoliosisCoach
@PilatesSportsCenter @PSCPilates @WellnessCenterofEncino

Contact Dr Stevens, DC:
www.ScoliosisCoach.com
ScoliosisCoach@gmail.com
https://linktr.ee/scoliosiscoach

Other Publications by Dr. Stevens, DC:
https://sites.google.com/view/future-general-
entertainement/home

ABBREVIATIONS / DEFINITIONS / TERMINOLOGY:

3-D correction: The correction of the body in all three anatomical planes. This involves correction of the coronal plane deformities (i.e., thoracic and lumbar curves), transverse
plane deformities (i.e., pelvic torsion and thoracic rotation) and sagittal plane deformities (i.e., hyperkyphosis). The objective is that the correction occurs simultaneously in three planes of space, as a unique movement called torsion and not plane-by-plane correction.

A.
Activities of Daily Living (ADLs):
The things normally done in daily living including any
daily activity performed for self-care (eating, bathing, dressing, grooming), work, homemaking and leisure.

Adams Forward Bend Test: A test is used to screen for scoliosis and to measure in degrees the amount of rotation associated with a scoliotic curve.

Adolescent scoliosis: A lateral spinal curvature that appears around puberty and before skeletal maturity, typically between 10-14 years old.

Adult scoliosis: Scoliosis that presents after skeletal maturity.

Allograft Bone: Bone that is taken from one individual, sterilized and available for use in a patient needing surgical fusion.

Anterior: The front

Anteroposterior view (AP view): An image view taken from the front of the body to the back (anterior to posterior)

Apex of the curve or Apical vertebra: The vertebra that is located at the farthest point out laterally from the midline of the body (convex side).

Apical vertebra – The vertebra the greatest distance from the midline with the most rotation

Apophysis: A growth plate that is used to estimate a child's skeletal maturity.

Atlas: the first cervical vertebra (C1) between the skull and the axis (C2).

Autogenous (or Autologous) Bone: Bone removed from one location in an individual and placed in a different location in the same individual (Pelvis, rib graft, or portions of the spinal bones can be used to assist with fusion).

Acronyms:
AIS: Adolescent idiopathic scoliosis
AAOS: American Academy of Orthopedic Surgeons
AAP: American Academy of Pediatrics
ART: Asymmetrical, Rigid, Torsion
ARV: Angle Reduction Velocity
ATR: Angle Trunk Rotation
ATSI: Anterior Trunk Symmetry Index

B.
Balanced curves: Scoliosis is referred to as balanced when two curves are approximately the same Cobb angle and have a more balanced appearance.

BCSG: Brace Classification Study Group

BRACE MAP: Building, Rigidity, Anatomical classification, Construction of the Envelope, Mechanism of Action, Plane of action

BMI: Body Mass Index

Bone Graft: bone (allograft or autologous) that is placed over implants or between other bones in a fusion.

BrAIST: Bracing in Adolescent Idiopathic Scoliosis Trial

C.
CAD/CAM: The term is an acronym defined as Computer-Aided Design/Computer-Aided Manufacturing. The process of making a shape capture with 3D modeling tools and a milling machine for fabrication.

Cervical spine: The seven bones (C1-C7) of the neck, The normal sagittal curve of the cervical spine is called lordosis.

Cobb angle: The universal standard of measurement used to determine the angle of scoliosis.

Coccyx: Also known as the tailbone.

Compensatory curve: a secondary curvature located above or below the major curve. This curve develops in an attempt to maintain normal body alignment.

Concave: A surface that curves inward.
Congenital scoliosis: Caused by bony abnormalities of the spine at birth.

Compliance: The degree of agreement between the patient's behavior and the recommendations of health professionals.

Convex: A surface that curves outward.

Corpectomy: Surgical removal of all or part of a vertebral body, also called a vertebral column resection or VCR.

CPO: Certified Prosthetic and Orthotic professional

CTLSO: Cervical-Thoraco-Lumbo-Sacral Orthotics

D.
Decompression: To relieve pressure on the spinal cord or nerve roots.

Deflexion (side-shift): Correction in the frontal plane of the ribs to the side.

Derotation: Correction in the transverse plane; twisting.

Dextroscoliosis: Curvature that goes to the right.

Disc: A soft, fluid-filled cartilage section between each vertebra that allows for absorption of loads and flexibility of the spine.

Disc degeneration: The loss of fluid, structure and functional integrity of an intervertebral disc.

Distal: Away from, or farthest from.

Dorsal: Posterior aspect, back.

Dorsal prominence: A "bump" on the back.

228

Double curve: Two side-to-side lateral curvatures in scoliosis.

Double major curve: Scoliosis in which there are two structural curves usually of equal or similar size.

Double thoracic curve: Two curves, both in the thoracic spine.

DRCS: Double Rib Contour Sign.

Dekyphotization: The action of reduction of the kyphosis of the spine.

Delordosization: The action of reducing the lordosis of the spine.

E.
EOS: Early-onset idiopathic scoliosis.

F.
Facet Joint: Laterally located joints between individual vertebrae that allow for movement, sometimes removed and used as a supplementary bone graft.

Flat Back Syndrome: A flattened upper (thoracic) or lower (lumbar) spine created by surgery, degeneration, or bracing.

Frontal plane: See: Planes of movement.

H.
Hyperkyphosis: A sagittal (front to back) alignment of the spine in which there is more than the normal amount of outward/backward bend.

Hypokyphosis: A sagittal (front to back) alignment of the spine in which there is less than the normal amount of outward/backward bend.

Hyperlordosis: A sagittal (front to back) alignment of the spine in which there is more than the normal amount of inward/ forward bend.

Hypolordosis: A sagittal (front to back) alignment of the spine in which there is less than the normal amount of inward/ forward bend.

Hemivertebra: A congenital abnormality of a bone caused by incomplete development into a wedge shape. This may cause scoliosis or kyphosis.

I.
IS: Idiopathic Scoliosis is structural spinal curvature with no known cause. Confirmed by X-ray. There are no underlying physical reasons for the curve. The most common type of scoliosis.

IBC: In-brace correction (IBC) is defined as the percentage of correction of all measurable parameters in all three body planes (frontal, sagittal, transverse) and the Cobb angle reduction during an X-ray with the brace fitted on the patient.

Iliac bone: The pelvic bone above the hip joint.
Infantile scoliosis: scoliosis that develops before three years of age.

Internal Fixation or Instrumentation: Immobilization of the mobile segments of the spine with implants to promote correction and fusion of these segments (an internal brace).

Intervertebral disc: Cartilage structure between two spinal vertebrae.

J.
Juvenile scoliosis: Scoliosis that develops between 3-10 years of age.

K.
Kyphoscoliosis: Structural scoliosis with an increased kyphosis resulting in a round-back appearance.

Kyphosis/kyphotic: The normal forward curvature of the spine front to back in the thoracic spine.

L.
Lateral: Away from the midline of the body.

Levoscoliosis: Scoliosis curvature to the left.

Lordoscoliosis: Scoliosis with increased lordosis in the low back.

Lordosis/lordotic: The normal alignment in the sagittal plane of the low back (lumbar) and the neck (cervical).

Lumbar curve: When the apex of the curve is between the 2-4th lumbar vertebrae.

Lumbar spine: Low back consisting of five large bones (L1 to L5) holding most of the body's weight.

Lumbosacral curve: Scoliosis with the apex of the curve at the 5th lumbar vertebra or lower.

LLD: Leg length discrepancy.

LSO: Lumbosacral orthosis.

M.
Major curve: Curvature with the largest Cobb angle.

Medial: Closer to the midline of the body.

Menarche: Menstrual period onset.

Mild scoliosis: 10º-24º degree Cobb angle measurement.

Mobilizations: Movements performed by oneself.

Moderate scoliosis: 25º – 49º degree Cobb angle measurement.

N.
Neuromuscular scoliosis: Scoliosis caused by a neurologic disorder.

Nonstructural curve (functional): Spinal curvature or scoliosis that is not fixed.

Non-progressive curve or scoliosis: A scoliotic curve in which the Cobb angle does not increase 5° or more during a six-month period.

O.
Osteotomy: A cut in a bone.

OTC: Open triradiate cartilage.

P.
PASB: Progressive Action Short Brace.

Pedicle: Part of the vertebra, shaped like an arch that connects the anterior and posterior segments of each vertebra.

Pedicle Screw: Screw placed posteriorly across the pedicle into the anterior part of the vertebral body, used as an anchor for a spinal rod.

PE: Polyethylene

POSNA: Pediatric Society of North America.

PSSE: Physiotherapeutic Scoliosis-Specific Exercises.

POTSI: Posterior Trunk Symmetry Index.

PP: Polypropylene

Positive mold: A solid mold formed from filling the negative cast with plaster.

Progressive curve or scoliosis: A scoliotic curve in which the Cobb angle increases 5° or more during a six-month period. Progression is also considered to be a sustained increase if the Cobb angle increases by at least 10°.

Passive movement: Movement aided by another person.

Planes of movement: Frontal/Sagittal: divides the body into left and right halves and the movement is front to back.

Median/Coronal: divides the body into front and back halves and the movement is lateral. Transverse: divides the body into top-to-bottom halves and the moment is rotational/twisting.

Posterior: In the back.

Primary curve: The first curve to appear when scoliosis becomes evident, also the first curve a human spine takes in development. Kyphosis is a primary curve, it came first.

Proximal: Closest

R.
RCB: Rigo Cheneau Brace.

RCT: Randomized Controlled Trial.

Re-kyphosis: Correction of the hypokyphosis by returning the vertebral column in the thoracic region to the normal physiological kyphosis of the sagittal plane.

Rib hump/bump: Ribs protrude backward due to rotation of the spine.

Risser Sign: A measurement from an X-ray used to evaluate skeletal maturity based on the pelvic apophysis. Graded from 0-5.

S.
Sacral spine/sacrum: Curved triangular bone at the base of the spine.

Sacroiliac joint (SI joint): Between the ilium and sacrum, there are two sides.

Sagittal plane: See: Planes of movement.

Schroth Method: A non-surgical, conservative approach to managing scoliosis. The techniques, developed in Germany, circa

1920, by Katharina Schroth, consist of specific exercises and breathing techniques.

Scoliometer: A measuring device used to measure rotations in the spine.

Secondary curve (compensatory): Develops in response to the major curve to try and help the body maintain alignment.

Self-elongation: Lengthening of the spine by yourself.

Severe scoliosis: Cobb angle measurement at or more than 50º.

Skeletal maturity: The Risser sign is graded 5 when measured on X-ray.

Spinous process: Vertebrae that protrude back from the spine create bumps when you bend over from the waist.

Structural curve: Segment(s) with a non-flexible curvature.

Symmetric spine: Appears to be equal or even on both sides.

Sagittal plane normalization: Sagittal plane correction. Obtaining a normal physiological kyphotic curve in the thoracic region as well as a normal physiological lordotic curve in the lumbar region, while maintaining the transition points of these regions.

SRS: Scoliosis Research Society.

SEAS: Scientific Exercises Approach to Scoliosis.

SOSORT: Society on Scoliosis Orthopedic and Rehabilitation Treatment.

SPoRT: Symmetrical, Patient-Oriented, Rigid, Three-Dimensional brace.

SRS: Scoliosis Research Society.

T.
TLSO: Thoraco-Lumbo-Sacral Orthosis.

Thoracic (Dorsal) spine: (T1-T12) including the 12 ribs.

Thoracic curvature: Apex of curvature is between the 2nd-11th thoracic vertebrae.

Thoracolumbar curve: Apex at the 12th thoracic or 1st lumbar vertebra.

Thoracolumbosacral Orthosis (TLSO): Type of back brace that immobilizes the thoracic, lumbar and sacral spine. This type of brace is used to attempt to prevent the progression of scoliosis curve(s) while a child/adolescent is in the growth phase.

Transverse plane: See: Planes of movement.

V.
Ventral flatzone: Flattening in the front rib cage.

Ventral prominence: Rib protrusion in the front of the body.

Vertebra: The 33 bones of the spinal column.

Vertebrae: Plural of the above.

Vertebral column: The 33 bones of the spine separated by discs.

EPILOGUE

I thought it was time to write down the basics whether you are a person with scoliosis or a parent trying to help your child navigate this confusing new landscape. My sincere hope is that my experience and knowledge will help any of you with your situation. I practice in Los Angeles and I welcome the chance to work with you or hear from you. Be well!

SCOLIOSIS SCREENING

Name:_____

Date: _____

Standing / Scoliometer Degrees:

Upper Back Curve: Right or Left: _____

Lower Back Curve: Right or Left: _____

Shoulder Forward: Right or Left: _____

Sagittal (front to back) Curves: _____

Notes / Questions:

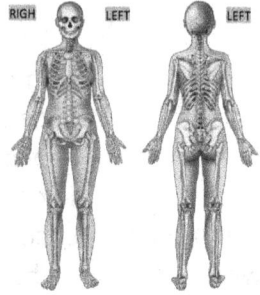

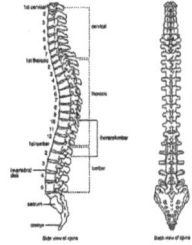

Draw curves or rib bumps on illustrations

AREA	ALIGNMENT SHOWS	STRATEGY NEEDED
Neck/Head tilt		
Right Shoulder Left Shoulder *Rotated or elevated?*		
Thoracic & Ribs Posterior View Lateral View		
Lumbar Posterior View Lateral View		
Pelvis Tiled, rotated or shifted		
Areas of Pain		
Notes:		

RESEARCH

Acupuncture
The effectiveness and safety of acupuncture for scoliosis: A protocol for systematic review and/or meta-analysis, by Choi SK, Jo HR, Park SH, Sung WS, Keum DH, Kim EJ. Medicine (Baltimore). 2020 Dec 11;99(50):e23238. doi: 10.1097/MD.0000000000023238. PMID: 33327244; PMCID: PMC7738006.
https://www.ncbi.nlm.nih.gov/pmc/articles/PMC7738006/

Bracing
Evaluation of the efficiency of Boston brace on scoliotic curve control: A review of literature, by Karimi MT, Rabczuk T.. J Spinal Cord Med. 2020 Nov;43(6):824-831. doi: 10.1080/10790268.2019.1578104. Epub 2019 Feb 27. PMID: 30811316; PMCID: PMC7808318.
https://www.ncbi.nlm.nih.gov/pmc/articles/PMC7808318/

Efficacy of the symmetric, patient-oriented, rigid, three-dimensional, active (SPoRT) concept of bracing for scoliosis: a prospective study of the Sforzesco versus Lyon brace, by Negrini S, Marchini G. Eura Medicophys. 2007 Jun;43(2):171-81; discussion 183-4. Epub 2006 Sep 24. PMID: 16955065.
https://pubmed.ncbi.nlm.nih.gov/16955065/

SOSORT Award Winner 2015: a multicentre study comparing the SPoRT and ART braces effectiveness according to the SOSORT-SRS recommendations, by Zaina, F., de Mauroy, J.C., Donzelli, S. *et al. Scoliosis* **10**, 23 (2015). https://doi.org/10.1186/s13013-015-0049-4
https://scoliosisjournal.biomedcentral.com/articles/10.1186/s13013-015-0049-4

240

The new Lyon ARTbrace versus the historical Lyon brace: a prospective case series of 148 consecutive scoliosis with short time results after 1 year compared with a historical retrospective case series of 100 consecutive scoliosis; SOSORT award winner 2015, by de Mauroy JC, Journe A, Gagaliano F, Lecante C, Barral F, Pourret S. winner. Scoliosis. 2015 Aug 19;10:26. doi: 10.1186/s13013-015-0047-6. PMID: 26300954; PMCID: PMC4545553.
https://www.ncbi.nlm.nih.gov/pmc/articles/PMC4545553/

Treatment of thoraco-lumbar curves in adolescent females affected by idiopathic scoliosis with a progressive action short brace (PASB): assessment of results according to the SRS committee on bracing and nonoperative management standardization criteria, by Aulisa AG, Guzzanti V, Galli M, Perisano C, Falciglia F, Aulisa L. Scoliosis. 2009 Sep 18;4:21. doi: 10.1186/1748-7161-4-21. PMID: 19765288; PMCID: PMC2754424.
https://pubmed.ncbi.nlm.nih.gov/19765288/

"Brace technology" thematic series - the Gensingen brace™ in the treatment of scoliosis, by Weiss HR. Scoliosis. 2010 Oct 13;5:22. doi: 10.1186/1748-7161-5-22. PMID: 20942970; PMCID: PMC2967515.
https://www.ncbi.nlm.nih.gov/pmc/articles/PMC2967515/
Incidentally, this is the brace that I recommend for my patients.

Factors associated with the success of the Rigo System Chêneau brace in treating mild to moderate adolescent idiopathic scoliosis, by Ovadia D, Eylon S, Mashiah A, Wientroub S, Lebel ED.. J Child Orthop. 2012 Aug;6(4):327-31. doi: 10.1007/s11832-012-0429-8. Epub 2012 Aug 14. PMID: 23904900; PMCID: PMC3425705.
https://pubmed.ncbi.nlm.nih.gov/23904900/

Effects of bracing in adolescents with idiopathic scoliosis, by Weinstein SL, Dolan LA, Wright JG, Dobbs MB. N Engl J Med. 2013 Oct 17;369(16):1512-21. doi: 10.1056/NEJMoa1307337. Epub 2013 Sep 19. PMID: 24047455; PMCID: PMC3913566.
https://pubmed.ncbi.nlm.nih.gov/24047455/

Bracing Rigid Vs. Soft Brace
Adolescent idiopathic scoliosis: indications for bracing and conservative treatments, by Kaelin AJ. Ann Transl Med. 2020 Jan;8(2):28. doi: 10.21037/atm.2019.09.69. PMID: 32055619; PMCID: PMC6995912.
https://www.ncbi.nlm.nih.gov/pmc/articles/PMC6995912/

Bracing In The Treatment Of Adolescent Idiopathic Scoliosis: Evidence To Date, by Karavidas N. Adolesc Health Med Ther. 2019 Oct 8;10:153-172. doi: 10.2147/AHMT.S190565. PMID: 31632169; PMCID: PMC6790111.
https://www.ncbi.nlm.nih.gov/pmc/articles/PMC6790111/

Bracing In The Treatment Of Adolescent Idiopathic Scoliosis: Evidence To Date, by Karavidas N. Adolesc Health Med Ther. 2019 Oct 8;10:153-172. doi: 10.2147/AHMT.S190565. PMID: 31632169; PMCID: PMC6790111.
https://www.ncbi.nlm.nih.gov/pmc/articles/PMC6790111/

Difference between Spinecor brace and Thoracolumbosacral orthosis for deformity correction and quality of life in adolescent idiopathic scoliosis, by Ersen O, Bilgic S, Koca K, Ege T, Oguz E, Bilekli AB.. Acta Orthop Belg. 2016 Dec;82(4):710-714. PMID: 29182110.
https://pubmed.ncbi.nlm.nih.gov/29182110/

Bracing and Congenital Scoliosis

Congenital Scoliosis (Mini-review), by Weiss HR, Moramarco M.. Curr Pediatr Rev. 2016;12(1):43-7. doi: 10.2174/1573396312666151117121011. PMID: 26769614.
https://pubmed.ncbi.nlm.nih.gov/26769614/

Conservative Treatment of Congenital Scoliosis, by Hans-Rudolf Weiss and Deborah Turnbull
Open Orthopedics Journal 2019, Volume: 13 Publisher ID: TOORTHJ-13-8 DOI: 10.2174/1874325001913010008
https://openorthopaedicsjournal.com/VOLUME/13/PAGE/8/

Congenital scoliosis – presentation of three severe cases treated conservatively, by H.R. Weiss
DOI 10.3233/978-1-58603-888-5-310 Series Studies in Health Technology and Informatics Ebook Volume 140: Research into Spinal Deformities 6
https://ebooks.iospress.nl/volumearticle/11871

Wedged vertebrae normalization in congenital scoliosis due to application of external forces by brace, by Chêneau, J., Grivas, T.B., Engels, G. *et al.* Scoliosis 2 (Suppl 1), S29 (2007).
https://doi.org/10.1186/1748-7161-2-S1-S29
https://link.springer.com/article/10.1186/1748-7161-2-S1-S29

Bracing Combined with Scoliosis-Specific Postural Exercise

The effectiveness of combined bracing and exercise in adolescent idiopathic scoliosis based on SRS and SOSORT criteria: a prospective study, by Negrini S, Donzelli S, Lusini M, Minnella S, Zaina F.. BMC Musculoskelet Disord. 2014 Aug 6;15:263. doi: 10.1186/1471-2474-15-263. PMID: 25095800; PMCID: PMC4132192.
https://pubmed.ncbi.nlm.nih.gov/25095800/

2016 SOSORT guidelines: orthopaedic and rehabilitation treatment of idiopathic scoliosis during growth, by Negrini, S., Donzelli, S., Aulisa, A.G. *et al. Scoliosis* **13**, 3 (2018). https://doi.org/10.1186/s13013-017-0145-8 https://scoliosisjournal.biomedcentral.com/articles/10.1186/s13013-017-0145-8#citeas

The effect of Schroth exercises added to the standard of care on the quality of life and muscle endurance in adolescents with idiopathic scoliosis-an assessor and statistician blinded randomized controlled trial: "SOSORT 2015 Award Winner," by Schreiber S, Parent EC, Moez EK, Hedden DM, Hill D, Moreau MJ, Lou E, Watkins EM, Southon SC. Scoliosis. 2015 Sep 18;10:24. doi: 10.1186/s13013-015-0048-5. PMID: 26413145; PMCID: PMC4582716. https://pubmed.ncbi.nlm.nih.gov/26413145/

Whether Orthotic Management and Exercise are Equally Effective to the Patients With Adolescent Idiopathic Scoliosis in Mainland China?: A Randomized Controlled Trial Study, by Zheng Y, Dang Y, Yang Y, Li H, Zhang L, Lou EHM, He C, Wong M. Spine (Phila Pa 1976). 2018 May 1;43(9):E494-E503. doi: 10.1097/BRS.0000000000002412. Erratum in: Spine (Phila Pa 1976). 2020 Sep 15;45(18):E1215. PMID: 28885287. https://pubmed.ncbi.nlm.nih.gov/28885287/

The efficacy of Schroth exercises combined with the Chêneau brace for the treatment of adolescent idiopathic scoliosis: a retrospective controlled study, by Fang MQ, Huang XL, Wang W, Li YA, Xiang GH, Yan GK, Ke CR, Mao CH, Wu ZY, Pan TL, Zhu RB, Xiao J, Yi XH. Disabil Rehabil. 2022 Sep;44(18):5060-5068. doi: 10.1080/09638288.2021.1922521. Epub 2021 May 13. PMID: 33984249. https://pubmed.ncbi.nlm.nih.gov/33984249/

CBD

What is Cannabidiol (CBD)
https://medlineplus.gov/druginfo/natural/1439.html

Consumer Update on Cannabis U.S National Library of Medicine, November 13, 2019, accessed February 6, 2020.
https://www.fda.gov/consumers/consumer-updates/what-you-need-know-and-what-were-working-find-out-about-products-containing-cannabis-or-cannabis

FDA Approval of drug derived from marijuana U.S. Food & Drug Administration, June 25, 2018.
https://www.fda.gov/news-events/press-announcements/fda-approves-first-drug-comprised-active-ingredient-derived-marijuana-treat-rare-severe-forms

FDA on cannabis and CDB during pregnancy
U.S. Food & Drug Administration, accessed March 16, 2020.
https://www.fda.gov/consumers/consumer-updates/what-you-should-know-about-using-cannabis-including-cbd-when-pregnant-or-breastfeeding

Genetics

Adolescent idiopathic scoliosis and genetic testing, by Ogilvie J. Adolescent idiopathic scoliosis and genetic testing. Curr Opin Pediatr. 2010 Feb;22(1):67-70. doi: 10.1097/MOP.0b013e32833419ac. PMID: 19949338.
https://pubmed.ncbi.nlm.nih.gov/19949338/

A Genetic Test Predicts Providence Brace Success for Adolescent Idiopathic Scoliosis When Failure Is Defined as Progression to >45 Degrees, by Bohl DD, Telles CJ, Ruiz FK, Badrinath R, DeLuca PA, Grauer JN. Clin Spine Surg. 2016 Apr;29(3):E146-50. doi: 10.1097/BSD.0b013e3182aa4ce1. PMID: 27007790.
https://pubmed.ncbi.nlm.nih.gov/27007790/

Epigenetic and Genetic Factors Related to Curve Progression in Adolescent Idiopathic Scoliosis: A Systematic Scoping Review of the Current Literature, by Faldini C, Manzetti M, Neri S, Barile F, Viroli G, Geraci G, Ursini F, Ruffilli A. Int J Mol Sci. 2022 May 25;23(11):5914. doi: 10.3390/ijms23115914. PMID: 35682604; PMCID: PMC9180299.
https://pubmed.ncbi.nlm.nih.gov/30774488/

Hormones
Does hormone replacement therapy prevent lateral rotatory spondylolisthesis in postmenopausal women? by Marty-Poumarat C, Ostertag A, Baudoin C, Marpeau M, de Vernejoul MC, Cohen-Solal M. Eur Spine J. 2012 Jun;21(6):1127-34. doi: 10.1007/s00586-011-2048-3. Epub 2011 Oct 28. PMID: 22033571; PMCID: PMC3366144.
https://www.ncbi.nlm.nih.gov/pubmed/22033571

Melatonin
Could long-term administration of melatonin to prepubertal children affect timing of puberty? By Boafo A, Greenham S, Alenezi S, Robillard R, Pajer K, Tavakoli P, De Koninck J. Nat Sci Sleep. 2019 Jan 31;11:1-10. doi: 10.2147/NSS.S181365. PMID: 30774488; PMCID: PMC6362935.
https://pubmed.ncbi.nlm.nih.gov/30774488/

Pseudoarthrosis
Pseudarthrosis in primary fusions for adult idiopathic scoliosis: incidence, risk factors, and outcome analysis, by Kim YJ, Bridwell KH, Lenke LG, Rinella AS, Edwards C 2nd. Spine (Phila Pa 1976). 2005 Feb 15;30(4):468-74. doi: 10.1097/01.brs.0000153392.74639.ea. Erratum in: Spine. 2005 Apr 15;30(8):994. Edward, Charles 2nd [corrected to Edwards, Charles 2nd]. PMID: 15706346.
https://pubmed.ncbi.nlm.nih.gov/15706346/

Quality of Life After Surgery
Health-related quality-of-life in adolescent idiopathic scoliosis patients 25 years after treatment, by Simony, A., Hansen, E.J., Carreon, L.Y. *et al. Scoliosis* **10**, 22 (2015). https://doi.org/10.1186/s13013-015-0045-8
https://scoliosisjournal.biomedcentral.com/articles/10.1186/s13013-015-0045-8

Risser 4/Skeletal Maturity and Treating Scoliosis
The Risser classification: a classic tool for the clinician treating adolescent idiopathic scoliosis, by Hacquebord JH, Leopold SS. Clin Orthop Relat Res. 2012 Aug;470(8):2335-8.
https://www.ncbi.nlm.nih.gov/pmc/articles/PMC3392381/

Sagittal Plane and Scoliosis
Children's Hospital of Philadelphia study by Saba Pasha: *3D Deformation Patterns of S Shaped Elastic Rods as a Pathogenesis Model for Spinal Deformity in Adolescent Idiopathic Scoliosis*, now supports and expands upon previous publications regarding the sagittal plane, scoliosis and perhaps one explanation regarding the cause of scoliosis.

Scoliometer
Scoliometer measurements of patients with idiopathic scoliosis, by Coelho DM, Bonagamba GH, Oliveira AS.. Braz J Phys Ther. 2013 Mar-Apr;17(2):179-84. doi: 10.1590/S1413-35552012005000081. PMID: 23778766.
https://pubmed.ncbi.nlm.nih.gov/23778766/

Scoliosis Specific Postural Exercise Programs (SSPE) for Scoliosis
Exercises reduce the progression rate of adolescent idiopathic scoliosis: results of a comprehensive systematic review of the literature, by Negrini S, Fusco C, Minozzi S, Atanasio S, Zaina F, Romano M.. Disabil Rehabil. 2008;30(10):772-85. doi: 10.1080/09638280801889568. PMID: 18432435.
https://pubmed.ncbi.nlm.nih.gov/18432435/

The efficacy of Schroth 3-dimensional exercise therapy in the treatment of adolescent idiopathic scoliosis in Turkey, by Otman S, Kose N, Yakut Y. Saudi Med J. 2005 Sep;26(9):1429-35. PMID: 16155663.
https://pubmed.ncbi.nlm.nih.gov/16155663/

Skeletal Maturity/Curve Progression
Prediction of progression of the curve in girls who have adolescent idiopathic scoliosis of moderate severity, by Peterson LE, Nachemson AL. Logistic regression analysis based on data from The Brace Study of the Scoliosis Research Society. J Bone Joint Surg Am. 1995 Jun;77(6):823-7. doi: 10.2106/00004623-199506000-00002. PMID: 7782354.
https://pubmed.ncbi.nlm.nih.gov/7782354/

The prediction of curve progression in untreated idiopathic scoliosis during growth, by Lonstein JE, Carlson JM. J Bone Joint Surg Am. 1984 Sep;66(7):1061-71. PMID: 6480635.
https://pubmed.ncbi.nlm.nih.gov/6480635/

Progression risk of idiopathic juvenile scoliosis during pubertal growth, by Charles YP, Daures JP, de Rosa V, Diméglio A. Spine (Phila Pa 1976). 2006 Aug 1;31(17):1933-42. doi: 10.1097/01.brs.0000229230.68870.97. PMID: 16924210.
https://pubmed.ncbi.nlm.nih.gov/16924210/

Curve progression in idiopathic scoliosis, by Weinstein SL, Ponseti IV.. J Bone Joint Surg Am. 1983 Apr;65(4):447-55. PMID: 6833318.
https://pubmed.ncbi.nlm.nih.gov/6833318/

Natural history of untreated idiopathic scoliosis after skeletal maturity, by Ascani E, Bartolozzi P, Logroscino CA, Marchetti PG, Ponte A, Savini R, Travaglini F, Binazzi R, Di Silvestre M. Spine (Phila Pa 1976). 1986 Oct;11(8):784-9. doi: 10.1097/00007632-198610000-00007. PMID: 3810293.
https://pubmed.ncbi.nlm.nih.gov/3810293/

Surgery

Indication for surgical treatment in patients with adolescent Idiopathic Scoliosis – a critical appraisal, by Weiss, HR., Moramarco, M.. *Patient Saf Surg* 7, 17 (2013).
https://doi.org/10.1186/1754-9493-7-17

Radiographic outcomes of anterior spinal fusion versus posterior spinal fusion with thoracic pedicle screws for the treatment of Lenke Type I adolescent idiopathic scoliosis curves, by Potter BK, Kuklo TR, Lenke LG. Spine (Phila Pa 1976). 2005 Aug 15;30(16):1859-66. doi: 10.1097/01.brs.0000174118.72916.96. PMID: 16103856.
https://pubmed.ncbi.nlm.nih.gov/16103856/

X-ray / EOS / MRI

Imaging in the Diagnosis and Monitoring of Children with Idiopathic Scoliosis, by Ng SY, Bettany-Saltikov J.. Open Orthop J. 2017 Dec 29;11:1500-1520. doi: 10.2174/1874325001711011500. PMID: 29399226; PMCID: PMC5759132.
https://www.ncbi.nlm.nih.gov/pmc/articles/PMC5759132/

Radiation dose of digital radiography (DR) versus micro-dose x-ray (EOS) on patients with adolescent idiopathic scoliosis. Hui, S.C.N., Pialasse, JP., Wong, J.Y.H. *et al.* 2016 SOSORT- IRSSD "John Sevastic Award" Winner in Imaging Research. *Scoliosis* 11, 46 (2016). https://doi.org/10.1186/s13013-016-0106-7

INTERVIEW QUESTIONS

Surgeon/Orthopedist Questions

- What are the risks and benefits of having surgery now vs. not going ahead with surgery at this time? Is there any harm in waiting? Will my condition become worse if I do not have the surgery?
- How do I know if spinal surgery will help me?
- Am I too young or too old for spinal surgery?
- What else can be done to relieve my symptoms besides surgery?
- Why is this type of surgery recommended?

The actual surgery

- Are there different methods for doing this surgery?
- What will the surgery be like?
- What steps will be involved in this surgery?
- How long will the surgery last?
- What type of anesthesia will be used? Are there choices to consider?
- Will I have a tube connected to my bladder? If yes, how long does it stay in?
- What will my stay in the hospital be like?

Hospital

- Does it make a difference which hospital I go to? Do I have a choice of where to have surgery?
- How long will I stay in the hospital?
- Will I be able to go home after being in the hospital, or will I need to go to a rehabilitation facility to recover more?

- Cost/Insurance
- How much will surgery cost?
- How do I find out if my insurance will pay for spinal surgery?
- Does insurance cover all of the costs or just some of them?

Preparing

- What can I do before surgery to make the risks lower?
- Is there anything that I can do before the surgery so it will be more successful for me? Are there exercises I should do to make my muscles stronger first?
- Do I need to lose weight before surgery?
- How can I get my home ready before I go to the hospital?
- Do I need to stop taking any medicines before my surgery?
- Will I need a blood transfusion during or after the surgery?
- What should I do the night before my surgery?
- When do I need to stop eating or drinking?
- Do I need to use a special soap when I bathe or shower?
- What medicines should I take on the day of surgery?
- What should I bring with me to the hospital?

Post Surgery

- How much help will I need when I come home? Will I be able to get out of bed?
- What type of supplies will I need when I get home?
- Will I be in a lot of pain after surgery? What will be done to relieve the pain?
- How soon will I be getting up and moving around?
- How long will it take to recover from spinal surgery?

- How should I manage the side effects such as swelling, soreness, and pain after the surgery?

- How will I care for the wound and sutures at home?

- Are there any restrictions post-surgery?

- Do I need to wear any kind of brace after spinal surgery?

- How long will it take for my back to heal after the surgery?

- How will spinal surgery affect my work and routine activities?

- How long will I need to be off work after the surgery?

- When will I be able to resume my routine activities on my own?

- When can I resume my medicines? How long should I not take anti-inflammatory medications?

- How will I gain my strength back after the spinal surgery?

- Do I need a rehabilitation program or physical therapy after the surgery? How long will the program last?

- What type of exercises will be included in this program?

- Will I be able to perform any exercises on my own after the surgery?

Orthotist/Bracing Questions

- What type of brace design do you make?

- What type of brace design will be created for me and why is this design best for me?

- How long will it take to get my brace?

- What will be the schedule for wearing my new brace? Will I start slowly? What will be the goal in terms of hours per day?

- When will I need X-rays wearing the brace to see how well it is working?

- How will I put on my brace and will I need help?

- What activities can I do and what activities should I not do with my brace on?

- What can I wear under and over the brace?

- How will I coordinate my sports activities and time out of the brace? How will that impact the brace-wearing schedule?

- Is there any special care I need for the brace and how do I clean it?

- Will there be another visit to follow up and make any bracing adjustments?

- What happens if my brace needs to be repaired?

- What happens if I outgrow the brace or if it needs to be replaced?

www.ingramcontent.com/pod-product-compliance
Lightning Source LLC
Chambersburg PA
CBHW052124270326
41930CB00012B/2751